COMMUNICATION DISORDERS AND INTERVENTIONS IN LOW INCIDENCE PEDIATRIC POPULATIONS

COMMUNICATION DISORDERS AND INTERVENTIONS IN LOW INCIDENCE PEDIATRIC POPULATIONS

Lisa Schoenbrodt, Ed.D.
Loyola College in Maryland
Romayne A. Smith, M.A.
Private Practice

SINGULAR PUBLISHING GROUP
SAN DIEGO · LONDON

Singular Publishing Group, Inc.
4284 41st Street
San Diego, California 92105-1197

19 Compton Terrace
London, N1 2UN, UK

Typeset in 11/13 Palatino by So Cal Graphics
Printed in the United States of America by McNaughton & Gunn

Library of Congress Cataloging-in-Publication Data

Schoenbrodt, Lisa, 1961–
Communication disorders and interventions in low incidence pediatric populations / Lisa Schoenbrodt and Romayne A. Smith.
p. cm.
Includes bibliographical references and index
ISBN 1-56593-220-X
1. Communicative disorders in children. I. Smith, Romayne. II. Title.
[DNLM: 1. Communicative Disorders—in infancy & childhood. WL 340.2 S365c 1995]
RJ496.C67S36 1995
618.92'855—dc20
DNLM/DLC
for Library of Congress

95–5807
CIP

CONTENTS

FOREWORD

The scope of practice for speech-language pathologists has been expanding. We now work with infants, toddlers, children, and adolescents with a wide range of communication disorders. Low incidence pediatric populations are part of the caseload for many speech-language pathologists working in schools, developmental centers, hospitals, and private practice.

Low incidence does not mean low priority. If you are working with one child and his or her family, his or her needs and communication challenges are a high priority for you and the child's family. When a condition has a low incidence, however, it may mean that you do not have a great deal of information about the condition. The authors of this book have reviewed and gathered together current information on low incidence pediatric populations into a clinical reference manual.

Communication Disorders and Interventions in Low Incidence Pediatric Populations provides state-of-the-art information on the medical background and etiology, communication characteristics, assessment, intervention, and professional collaboration for a variety of conditions associated with communication disorders, including traumatic brain injury, attention deficit disorder, Tourette syndrome, Fragile X syndrome, neglect and abuse, prenatal drug exposure, and autism and pervasive developmental disorders.

Lisa Schoenbrodt and Romayne Smith have compiled information on each disorder that is helpful to practicing speech-language pathologists and included practical suggestions for intervention strategies. The information could also provide background on the communication needs and challenges of children with these low incidence disorders for special educators, teachers, psychologists, and other professionals who work with them. The information is well-organized and current. The book also could serve as a background text or reference text for graduate courses in language disorders of children.

Communication Disorders and Interventions in Low Incidence Pediatric Populations provides a needed source of information. The appendixes suggest resources for additional information about each low incidence pediatric problem area. We now have information on a wide variety of communication disorders in low incidence pediatric populations in one clinical reference.

Libby Kumin, Ph.D., CCC-SLP
Loyola College in Maryland

PREFACE

Professionals who focus on diagnosis and intervention with the pediatric population are continuously faced with new challenges. In schools, clinics, hospitals, and private practitioners' offices, children are being diagnosed with various disorders affecting communication. Many of these disorders statistically are on the rise due to factors and/or problems in society (e.g., child abuse/neglect, fetal alcohol syndrome, head injury, etc.); in other disorders, communication problems are just recently being recognized as a major deficit area.

Speech-language pathologists have the knowledge and expertise to provide accurate diagnosis and treatment of communication disorders. However, with recent changes of the scope of intervention services in schools to more inclusive practices and classroom-based instruction, all professionals—including teachers, special educators, psychologists, and others—must be educated in this area as well.

We have collaborated to write this book with the intention of providing a clinical reference tool that contains accurate, relevant, and as current as possible information regarding communication problems in low incidence pediatric populations. For several of the populations addressed in the book, little current information was available regarding intervention issues specific to communication disorders. This does not mean that, as speech-language pathologists or educators, we should not be intervening with these groups. The lack of information available simply highlights the great need for further research on intervention with these populations so that we may enhance our abilities as professionals to increase children's communication competence.

Throughout the book, the structure of the chapters is similar to allow readers to identify overlapping characteristics as well as contrasts among the various populations. References are provided for further reading in each area. In addition, appendixes identifying resources and support organizations for each population are included. We hope this book will encourage clinicians to delve deeper and experiment more with the best practices that are effective with the targeted populations.

ACKNOWLEDGMENTS

There are individuals we would like to acknowledge for their ideas, support, and encouragement.

We would like to express our appreciation to Marie Linvill of Singular Publishing Group for her support and continued patience during the writing of this book. We would also like to thank Ann Beetz, Robert Serianni, Danielle Dehn Matrangola, Clyde Robinette, Psy.D., Gwen Martinson, Ph.D., and Sue Okun for their tireless efforts in helping us with proofreading and editing and for giving us feedback on the contents of the book. Finally, we would like to express our gratitude to our families who extended their support and patience throughout the completion of the book: Scott, David, and Matthew Myers, Frederick and Margaret Schoenbrodt, and Clyde Robinette.

CHAPTER 1

Traumatic Brain Injury

Definition

According to the National Head Injury Foundation (1985), *traumatic brain injury* (TBI) is an insult to the brain, not of a degenerative or congenital nature, caused by an external physical force, that may produce a diminished or altered state of consciousness, which results in the impairment of cognitive abilities or physical functioning. A brain injury also can result in the disturbance of behavioral or emotional functioning. These impairments may be either temporary or permanent and cause partial or total functional disability or psychosocial maladjustment.

There are two major types of head injury: closed head injury and open head injury. In a closed head injury, the skull is not penetrated, and damage to the brain is more diffuse. Diffuse or generalized damage can occur anywhere in the brain and may cause variable behavior and learning problems for the child having a head injury. In an open head injury, the skull is penetrated, as in a gunshot wound, and the damage is localized to the site of penetration.

Incidence

TBI is the primary cause of death and disability in children today. Falls and abuse are the principle etiology of TBI in the preschool years. Children ages 5 to 14 are often injured in sports-related activities or pedestrian and bicycle accidents. Children over the age of 14 generally sustain a TBI as a result of motor vehicle accidents.

Epidemiological studies have shown age and gender to be important factors in determining who is at risk to suffer a TBI (Waaland & Cockrell, 1990). Boys are more likely to sustain a brain injury than girls. Adolescents are at the highest risk for brain injury, followed by preschoolers. In addition, children who have previously sustained a head injury are more likely to sustain another one.

Variables Associated with Outcome in TBI

Outcome of TBI is predicted by the degree and length of coma after the accident and the duration of post-traumatic amnesia (PTA). PTA is defined as the period of time which begins with the onset of coma and ends when the child can continuously remember. Other prognostic indicators include the child's premorbid level of health and pre-existing learning or educational problems (learning disability, attention deficit disorder, etc.).

Degree and Length of Coma

The *Glasgow Coma Scale* (GCS) (Jennett & Teasdale, 1981) and the *Rancho Los Amigos Levels of Cognitive Functioning Scale* (Hagen, 1986) are commonly used in assessing the child with a TBI. The GCS (Jennett & Teasdale, 1974) measures eye opening, motor, and verbal responses on a scale from 0 to 15. This scale is typically used in the hospital to evaluate the degree of severity of the head injury. A mild head injury would be defined as a GCS of 13 or better with either no loss of consciousness or loss of consciousness for less than 20 minutes. A moderate head injury is defined as a GCS of 8 to 12 with loss of consciousness for more than 20 minutes and an accompanying fracture with contusions. A severe head injury is defined as a GCS of 7 or less accompanied by intracranial hematoma, fracture with neurological deficit, bruising and contusion of brain tissue. The relationship between GCS scores and outcome has not been studied extensively in children with TBI, causing its predictive validity to be questioned (Lehr, 1989).

The validity of medical designations used to classify TBI has also been questioned, suggesting that the current classification system of mild, moderate, and severe may not be the best indicators of outcome or potential for school-related problems (Savage, 1991). The *Rancho Los Amigos Levels of Cognitive Functioning Scale* (Hagen, 1986) may be more appropriate to use for interpretation of the child's recovery because it assesses the child's progress during the rehabilitation process.

Age at Injury

The common assumption that infants, toddlers, and preschoolers are more resilient to TBI because of their age has not been supported. The immature skull is thinner and more easily damaged by trauma, has limited protective covering, and incomplete myelination. Young children are also more at risk for increased intracranial pressure, diffuse swelling, and secondary brain injuries.

In addition, the younger the child, the greater the long-term cognitive impairment is likely to be due to immature neuroanatomy and lack of formal learning. The pediatric TBI population is also unique in that there is the potential for delayed onset of deficits. There is evidence of increased risk of late seizure onset in children under 2 years of age. The injury can affect areas in the child's brain that are still developing and deficits may not be evident for years post-onset.

Characteristics of Children with TBI

The deficits following TBI can be present in one area or in combinations of areas including physical, cognitive, communicative, perceptual-motor, and psychosocial (see Table 1–1).

Assessment

An in-depth multidisciplinary evaluation of the child with a TBI is necessary to identify cognitive strengths and weaknesses, establish baseline behavior, and for litigation purposes.

Children who have sustained head injuries are each unique, and their cognitive, psychomotor and psychosocial profiles are unpredictable. Variability is evident throughout all stages of recovery. When conducting an evaluation, it is important to keep the child's premorbid level of functioning in mind as a mechanism for comparison in determining educational placement and support services.

Standardized testing is necessary to document comparable scores and eligibility for educational and support services. A formal assessment battery should evaluate functioning in the

Table 1–1. Types of deficits following TBI.

Area	Description
Physical	Difficulties in mobility, strength, coordination, vision, hearing, and seizure disorders.
Cognitive	Problems with memory, attention, concentration, judgment, processing of information and problem-solving skills; indecisive, distractible, confabulation, perseverative, rigid, and inflexible.
Communicative	Deficits in language, articulation, word-finding, reading, writing, and abstraction; metacognitive weaknesses.
Perceptual-Motor	Reduced speed of movement and eye-hand coordination; visual, auditory, and tactile deficits; spatial disorientation.
Psychosocial	Poor self-image and motivation; apathy, lack of inhibition, social withdrawal, depression, denial, aggressive behavior, dependency.

following areas: intellectual, executive, problem-solving, attention, concentration, memory, speech and language, perceptual-motor, and academic abilities. It is important for examiners to choose instruments that sample the full spectrum of cognitive processes. A list of assessments is provided in Appendix H).

The following general characteristics also should be observed during evaluation of the child with TBI: level of attention, tolerance to stress (time constraints, noise, frustration), degree of cuing and prompting necessary, utilization of compensatory strategies, processing time, delayed response, or slowed performance, anxiety, fear of failure, and fatigue. These factors should also be taken into consideration when administering an assessment. Fatigue is a common problem following a head injury. Assessments should be broken into several testing sessions according to the child's level of stamina. Visual field deficits are also common following a head trauma. Visual stimuli may need to be adapted by enlarging printed material or by altering the location of presentation (to the nonaffected side).

An in-depth evaluation should include an informal or naturalistic assessment. This type of assessment collects information about a child's performance through interviews, questionnaires, performance rating scales, and behavioral observations. The child should be observed in a variety of settings and contexts (e.g., in the gymnasium, cafeteria, playground, and classroom). For example, an observation of the child with a head injury in the cafeteria would yield information regarding his or her ability to process information in a noisy environment, communicative competence, ability to communicate under time constraints (in the lunch line), word finding difficulties, problem-solving difficulties, and so on. Such invaluable information is not provided by a standardized assessment. In fact, the information obtained on a standardized assessment may be deceiving. A student may obtain "average" scores on the administered assessments, but not be able to function appropriately at home or in the school environment. On the other hand, a child may function below average on many assessments, but be able to function adequately in daily life activities.

Evaluation of the child's pragmatic functions including conversational discourse and narratives is also important. These areas should be evaluated for the child's ability to maintain discourse and provide cohesion throughout a narrative. In addition, deficits may be evident in initiation, maintenance, turn-taking, repair, listening, and awareness of utterance duration (Russell, 1993). Frequently, children with head injuries exhibit pragmatic difficulties that affect discourse coherence, resulting in discourse that is fragmented, tangential, and irrelevant (Mentis & Prutting, 1991).

Because variability in performance is common in children having head injuries, ongoing assessment is important. Pretraumatic academic levels may be maintained, but difficulties often appear in the learning of new tasks. Continuing brain development also can complicate the ability to predict success.

Interpretation of Standardized Tests

Although standardized testing is important in the evaluation process, the clinician must remember that most instruments have not been normed using the head-injured population. Therefore, interpretation of scores should provide insight into the strengths and weaknesses of the student but should not be considered definitive.

Inconsistent performance is characteristic of children with head injuries. A child, for example, may not complete one-step directions accurately but will perform three-step directions with little difficulty. The variability in performance is important not only in interpretation of test results, but also in the administration of assessments. The evaluation should be administered in a standard manner. However, many subtests are timed or do not allow directions to be repeated. In these instances, the examiner should note the child's inability to complete the subtest in the standard fashion, but then should extend the time limits or repeat the directions to obtain additional information on the child's abilities.

Observation of a child's performance during the test-taking situation can yield information regarding the type of compensatory or cuing strategies the child uses. For example, if the child is given a task involving memory, it is important to note whether the child uses rehearsal or other strategies to retain the information. Memory deficits also can be observed in evaluation of pragmatic functions. A child having difficulty may not have the ability to recall information necessary to continue or repair a conversation. These deficits in turn may affect the child's ability to function effectively in social situations. These informal observations give more insight into developing a program for this child than does a test score.

Fatigue is also a common problem for children having head injuries. A child who does not complete various tasks may be viewed as lacking motivation and initiation, when in fact the fatigue is negatively affecting his or her performance. Administration of tests should be scheduled over several sessions. In addition, team members should coordinate the evaluation schedule so that the child is not overwhelmed.

In general, the results obtained from the standardized testing battery should be interpreted cautiously. The information obtained should be analyzed in terms of what the test purports to measure. A naturalistic assessment must be included as part of the formal battery of testing and should examine areas affecting both academic and nonacademic functioning (social skills). In completing and interpreting assessments, it is crucial to consider the pretraumatic skills of the student as well as the many post-traumatic deficits.

Treatment

Traumatic brain injury presents a number of deficits that interfere with the child's transition back to school: memory, behavior, emotion, attention, cognitive processing, concentration, intellectual deficits, and physical deficits. At the present time, few structured learning environments are available to serve only head-injured students. There are also no specific educational and language assessments designed to evaluate their deficits in learning.

Currently, barriers to meeting the needs of the student with a head injury are: (a) there is no tracking system of children having head injuries, and (b) special and regular education teachers have not been trained to recognize the resultant disabilities or in the methods necessary to help students with TBI. The biggest problem is the lack of information in school systems regarding children with head injuries.

With the recent reauthorization of Public Law (P.L.) 94-142 (1990), The Education of All Handicapped Children Act (P.L. 101-476), the committees of the United States Senate and House of Representatives supported the inclusion of the definition of TBI under the present category of "other health impaired." Inclusion of this definition was critical because it enables school districts to work with insurance companies to cover the cost of services for these students.

Inclusion of the definition of TBI in P.L. 101-476 also recognizes these students as having deficits that are different from other populations. Frequently, when children with head injuries returned to the school setting, they were placed in a classroom for learning disabled, mentally retarded, emotionally handicapped, and so on, when the deficits these children have are variable, not constant. However, even with the inclusion of TBI, many school systems generally recognize only students with severe head injuries. Students with moderate and mild head injuries often are not recognized, either because they have not been identified by the rehabilitation setting or because their needs are not understood by the educational setting (Savage, 1991).

In addition to the recent changes in the law, the rapid adoption of the ideas of "inclusion" and "collaborative consultation" in the classroom have changed the course of treatment strategies for children with head injuries. Students with severe head injuries still frequently receive services in self-contained classrooms. However, children with moderate to mild deficits may receive classroom-based communication services. For treatment to be effective, the speech-language pathologist should provide therapy in the classroom setting. Classroom-based communication services are provided in the natural environment and constraints in which the student has to function. This environment allows communication skills to be practiced under normally occurring circumstances. This type of practice is more meaningful to the student and allows for greater generalization of the learned skills to other environments.

The classroom-based communication model allows the speech-language pathologist to observe the types of learning contexts, learning styles (visual, auditory, etc.), educational requirements, environmental factors, as well as social contexts, in which the student has to perform. This model also allows the speech-language pathologist (SLP) and the classroom or special education teacher to consult together to form mutual goals for the student. For example, the teacher and SLP may consult to make unit plans focusing on the curriculum. The ideas they share can enhance classroom learning while considering the unique needs of the student with a head injury.

In addition, the recent focus of the whole language approach in schools also allows the SLP to be part of classroom-based therapy. The cognitive deficits that are apparent following a TBI frequently affect speaking, listening, reading, and writing which are areas targeted by the whole language approach. However, in many cases, the child's deficits are not severe enough to warrant speech and language services. Therefore, the collaboration between the SLP and the teacher in the whole language approach would benefit the student with TBI who does not qualify for services.

Classroom-based instruction also provides a natural environment for SLPs to observe and pursue social skills instruction. Many programs are available to provide practice and instruction in social skills. These programs focus on teaching or reteaching appropriate pragmatic skills in various social settings. For example, teaching the child how to initiate a conversation falls under the heading of "Friendship Making Skills." Social skills interventions often utilize role play as a means of practicing the skills. With the SLP involved in the classroom/school environment, students who have social skill deficits are able to practice these skills in a natural setting. Once again, the practice in a natural setting is more meaningful and promotes generalization of the skills to other environments like the cafeteria, playground, and eventually the community.

The above are only a few examples of the ways SLPs can be effective in providing classroom-based services for students with TBI. Certainly, there are students who need intensive individualized instruction due to severe language, cognitive, or behavioral deficits. Even in these cases, the SLP should consult with the classroom teacher to ensure successful reintegration of the learned skills to the classroom environment.

Case Management

In either setting, the speech-language pathologist is frequently sought as the case manager for the child with a head injury. The school speech-language pathologist should play an active role as part of the educational placement team in coordinating the student's transition from the rehabilitation setting to the school setting. Speech-language pathologists have knowledge of the neurological deficits and educational needs following a TBI which provides a foundation to act in the role of case manager (DePompei & Blosser, 1987; Russell, 1993).

The school speech-language pathologist should be in contact with the rehabilitation center before the student returns to school. Information should be obtained regarding the trauma, assessments that have been performed, severity of the injury, and initial impressions regarding outcome for the purpose of educational placement.

Additionally, educators and specialists who will be involved with the head-injured student when he or she returns to school should schedule a visit to the rehabilitation center while the student is there. Telephone contacts between the rehabilitation specialists and school personnel should be conducted frequently, even after the student returns to the school setting. Recent studies have shown that teachers list observations in the rehabilitation center followed by classroom training as ways to enhance their understanding of the needs of the head-injured student (Feeney & Urbanczyk, 1992). The rehabilitation staff should also be invited to the placement Annual Review and Dismissal/Individual Education Plan meeting to facilitate the transition process. Finally, the child's family should be involved in the transition to maintain ongoing communication about the student's skills, needs, and problems related to school re-entry.

One role of the speech-language pathologist as the case manager is to provide information to the child's teachers regarding the injury and the impact it can have on the student's functioning in the school environment. Information regarding the child's current level of performance in comparison to his or her premorbid performance should be presented. Educators also should be made aware of the differences between children having head injuries versus other types of disabilities, because children with head injuries frequently have characteristics similar to children with learning disabilities. However, basic differences are evident (Table 1–2).

One major difference is that the child's learning and communication deficits were acquired as a result of a traumatic injury. In many cases, the child had no learning difficulties prior to the trauma. Additional characteristics include:

1. A sense of being normal that persists from the premorbid period.
2. Discrepancies in ability levels.
3. A previous history of successful experiences in academic and social settings.
4. Inconsistent patterns of performance.
5. Variability and fluctuation in the recovery process, resulting in unpredictable and unexpected spurts of recovery.
6. More extreme problems with generalizing, integrating, or structuring information.
7. Poor judgment and loss of emotional control, which cause the student to appear emotionally disturbed at times.
8. Cognitive deficits that, although present in other handicaps, are more uneven in extent of damage and rate of recovery.
9. Combinations of handicapping conditions that do not fall into usual categories of disabilities.

Table 1–2. Similarities and differences in characteristics of children with traumatic brain injury (TBI) and children with learning disabilities LD).

Children with TBI	Children with LD
Acquired. Sudden onset.	Congenital deficit. Usually early onset.
Documented history of coma in many cases	No coma.
Cause attributed to event such as motor vehicle accident, gun shot wound, etc.	Cause not clear.
Documented post-traumatic amnesia (PTA) affecting memory.	Memory deficits not related to PTA.
Noticeable differences in premorbid skills and post trauma abilities.	No pre/post effect.
New learning difficult, can remember old skills.	Learning may be slow with continued progress in new learning.
Range of deficits from mild to severe	Range of deficits from mild to severe.
Poor social/pragmatic skills secondary to injury	Poor social/pragmatic skills secondary to language impairment.
Inability to comprehend post-traumatic deficits.	Good comprehension of learning strengths and weaknesses.
Seizure medications given for traumatically induced seizures.	No anti-seizure medication.
Marked impairment of progress initially indicating a need for frequent monitoring of progress. At the school level, annual review and	Slow, steady progress. Monitoring of progress may take place at the school level one or two times a year to document gains.

(continued)

Table 1–2. *(continued)*

Children with TBI	Children with LD
dismissal meetings should be held monthly until progress stabilizes.	
Once in school change of classroom placement may be needed when progress occurs.	Relatively stable. Classroom placement remains constant.
Needs modification in testing due to impairments (fatigue, distractibility, etc.) secondary to TBI.	Needs modification in testing due to impairments (distractibility, language deficits, etc.) of the LD.
Family may not accept child's school placement and needs due to problems coping with the deficits presented secondary to the sudden trauma.	Family generally understands strengths and weaknesses of child as well as the LD because onset was early and gradual.

10. Inappropriate behaviors that may be more exaggerated than the behaviors of students with other handicaps.
11. A learning style that requires the use of a variety of compensatory and adaptive strategies.
12. Some intact high-level skills which make it difficult to understand why the student has difficulties in performing lower level tasks.
13. A previously learned base of information that facilitates rapid learning. (Blosser & DePompei, 1989, p. 69)

The above information should be shared with the child's teachers so that they will be able to develop an awareness of the child's strengths and weaknesses and be able to program for the student in the classroom. In addition to educating teachers about traumatic brain injury, the speech-language pathologist should help teachers modify their means of instructing the head-injured student. DePompei and Blosser (1987, 1988) have suggested that the following modifications be incorporated by teachers of children with head injuries:

1. Accompany verbal instructions with written instructions and vice versa.
2. Avoid using figurative language.
3. Use pauses to direct the student's attention and allow time for processing.
4. Provide examples, pictures and written cues to illustrate important information and concepts.
5. Repeat instructions.
6. Redefine new words and terms.
7. Use concrete teaching materials, not abstract.
8. Maintain a structured environment.
9. Alert the student in advance to anticipated changes in the daily routine. (p. 71)

In addition to the above suggestions, teachers should be aware that the student may require a rest period during the school day due to physical fatigue or for emotional release. Requirements for class assignments may also need to be modified. Having a student complete all of the problems for an assignment may be fatiguing. One modification would be to reduce the number of questions to be answered. Other modifications include permitting the student to tape-record class lectures, changing the format of a test, or allowing the use of assistive devices such as calculators, tape recorders, and computers.

It is also imperative that the student be given help in formulating and using a system for maintaining organization. For example, keeping a daily planner, which includes space to record homework assignments, time of classes, and room, locker, and bus numbers, is important. It is equally important for teachers and specialists to monitor the child's use of the system daily.

As the case manager, the speech-language pathologist can provide the link for the student between the rehabilitation center to the school setting. The role of the case manager is important for several reasons: (a) to provide information to the educators who will be managing the student in the classroom setting; (b) to frequently monitor the progress of the student which may be variable due to constantly changing medical, behavioral, and cognitive deficits post-injury; (c) to act in conjunction with the monitoring of the student, making updates to the IEP, and enacting changes in placement due to the above variables; and (d) to act as a liaison for the student when the family is under emotional stress and may lack the jargon and knowledge necessary to act as an advocate for their child.

Family Issues

The family of the student with TBI plays an important role in facilitating the transition to the school and the community. As a result of the trauma, the family also experiences major alterations of roles, rules, and internal responsibilities in its adjustment to the affected family member.

The impact on the family of the child with a head injury begins with the telephone call informing them of the injury and continues through the rehabilitation process and a lifetime of outpatient care (DePompei & Zarski, 1989). Many studies have documented that all aspects of family life are affected by TBI and that major changes in structure and organization are inevitable. (Brooks, 1984; Prigatano & Klonoff, 1987; Rosenthal & Muir, 1983; Ylvisaker, Szekeres, Henry, Sullivan, & Wheeler, 1987)

Stress resulting from the changes in routine, social status, family health, and patient behaviors is a major factor in a family's ability to adjust to the family member with the head injury. In addition, the family of the person with the head injury has particular difficulty with the mourning process. This is because the family is unable to bury their loved one as when there is a death in the family (DePompei & Zarski, 1989). The person with the head injury remains with the family often in the same physical state but in an altered cognitive state.

The family must mourn the characteristics of the individual that have been lost while learning to respond to the differences in the person. The way in which a family responds is crucial in the outcome of the person with the head injury.

The functional family eventually draws internal and external support to respond to new needs of the family member and maintains hope for the future. A dysfunctional family is unable to focus on any factor other than the trauma and tends to concentrate on the weaknesses rather than the strengths of the individual.

Additionally, the family of a child who has TBI often is faced with overwhelming economic burdens in providing the long-term care that is required. For these reasons, it is crucial that the speech-language pathologist be involved directly with the family in communicating their needs to the educational team providing services to their child. As the case manager, the speech-language pathologist can act in a neutral role to serve the best interests of the head-injured student. For example, the family may be concerned about the inappropriate manner in which the head-injured child socializes with his or her siblings. The school can incorporate goals and objectives that address social skills which are necessary in the school, home, and community in the IEP.

Additionally, the family may be becoming increasingly aware of the medical outcome for their child, but lack knowledge about the educational system. Just as the family becomes somewhat accustomed to the jargon of the medical placement, they are faced with jargon like IEP, ARD, inclusion, and whole language. The speech-language pathologist can facilitate the child's transition to the school setting by explaining the laws, time lines, placement options, and the expectations of the school in terms of the development of goals and objectives.

Summary

The neurological and cognitive sequelae that result from head injury vary greatly in terms of severity across the population. For this reason, students with head injuries must be considered unique and treated on an individual basis.

With the implementation of the new disability category for brain injury mandated by P.L. 101-476, schools will need informed personnel to serve these students. The speech-language pathologist has a sound knowledge base about the neurological, cognitive, linguistic, behavioral, and educational factors that affect reintegration of students with TBI into the school setting. With this type of training, the speech-language pathologist is able to not only provide treatment, but also to act as case manager for the child's transition to the school setting.

CHAPTER 2

Attention Deficit Disorder

Definition

The term attention deficit disorder (ADD) was originally proposed by the American Psychiatric Association (APA) (1980) as a substitute for the term minimal brain dysfunction (APA, 1980). The terminology was changed to attention deficit hyperactivity disorder (ADHD) in 1987 (APA, 1987). Medical researchers used the term minimal brain dysfunction to include a cluster of symptoms including specific learning deficits, hyperkinesis, impulsivity, and short attention span as confirmed by examination of equivocal neurological signs and borderline abnormal or an abnormal electroencephalogram (EEG). The medical model focused on biological deficits, whereas educational researchers focused on academic and language difficulties and characterized children as having a learning disability.

The publication of the third edition of the *Diagnostic and Statistical Manual of Mental Disorders* (DSM-III) in 1987 represented a significant advance in the establishment of a valid diagnosis of hyperactivity (ADD). The term ADD was developed because investigators believed that attentional factors, rather than activity levels, were the major symptoms of the disorder (Cantwell, 1983; Douglas & Peters, 1979). DSM-III differentiated between two subtypes of ADD based on the presence or absence of symptoms of hyperactivity. However, no clear distinctions were made regarding the two subtypes: attention deficit disorder with hyperactivity (ADHD) and attention deficit disorder without hyperactivity (Epstein, Shaywitz, Shaywitz, & Woolston, 1991). DSM-III-R (1987) added further confusion to the differentiation. It focused on ADHD and classified attention deficit without hyperactivity in the category of undifferentiated ADD.

The diagnostic criteria for attention deficit with hyperactivity disorder of the DSM-IV (APA, 1994) include:

A. Either (1) or (2):
   (1) six (or more) of the following symptoms of inattention have persisted for at least 6 months to a degree that is maladaptive and inconsistent with developmental level:
   Inattention
   a. often fails to give close attention to details or makes careless mistakes in schoolwork, work, or other activities
   b. often has difficulty sustaining attention in tasks or play activities
   c. often does not seem to listen when spoken to directly
   d. often does not follow through on instructions and fails to finish schoolwork, chores, or duties in the workplace (not due to oppositional behavior or failure to understand instructions)
   e. often has difficulty organizing tasks and activities

f. often avoids, dislikes, or is reluctant to engage in tasks that require sustained mental effort (such as schoolwork or homework)
g. often loses things necessary for tasks or activities (e.g., toys, school assignments, pencils, books, or tools)
h. is often easily distracted by extraneous stimuli
i. is often forgetful in daily activities

(2) Six (or more) of the following symptoms of hyperactivity-impulsivity have persisted for at least six months to a degree that is maladaptive and inconsistent with developmental level:

Hyperactivity

a. often fidgets with hands or feet or squirms in seat
b. often leaves seat in classroom or in other situations in which remaining seated is expected
c. often runs about or climbs excessively in situations in which it is inappropriate (in adolescents or adults, may be limited to subjective feelings of restlessness)
d. often has difficulty playing or engaging in leisure activities quietly
e. is often "on the go" or often acts as if "driven by a motor"
f. often talks excessively

Impulsivity

g. often blurts out answers before questions have been completed
h. often has difficulty awaiting turn
i. often interrupts or intrudes on others (e.g., butts into conversations or games)

B. Some hyperactive-impulsive or inattentive symptoms that caused impairment were present before age seven years.

C. Some impairment from the symptoms is present in two or more settings (e.g., at school [or work] and at home).

D. There must be clear evidence of clinically significant impairment in social, academic, or occupational functioning.

E. The symptoms do not occur exclusively during the course of a Pervasive Developmental Disorder, Schizophrenia, or other Psychotic Disorder and are not better accounted for by another mental disorder. (e.g., Mood Disorder, Anxiety Disorder, Dissociative Disorder, or a Personality Disorder)(pp. 83–85)

DSM-IV (APA, 1994) presents separate criteria for ADHD and attention deficit disorder without hyperactivity (ADDnoH). Lahey and Carlson (1991) reported that the differentiation of these two syndromes of attention deficit disorder is supported by factor analysis studies which describe maladjustment in terms of (a) inattention and disorganization and (b) motor hyperactivity and impulsive responding. In comparison to children with ADHD, clinic-referred children with ADDnoH showed less serious conduct problems, were less impulsive, appeared more sluggish, were more withdrawn socially (but not rejected by their peers), and were more likely to exhibit symptoms of anxiety disorder. However, in most cases, it is the presence of hyperactivity or other behavioral symptomatology that serves as the major criterion for the provision of special education services.

In order for a child to be diagnosed as ADHD under DSM-III conditions, three specific criteria must be met. First, symptoms in the dimensions of inattention, impulsivity, and motor hyperactivity must exist. Second, the age of onset must be prior to 7 years of age. Third, the duration of these characteristics must be at least 6 months (APA, 1980). In contrast, for a child to be diagnosed ADHD with the DSM-III-R criteria (APA, 1987), any 8 to a possible 14 symptoms must be seen. As a result, more children now meet the criteria for ADHD and receive services under the present federal guidelines (Cantwell & Baker, 1991).

Incidence

Szatmari, Offord, and Boyle (1989) identified 11 studies reporting prevalence rates of ADHD. Among the 11 studies, prevalence rates varied from less than 1% to 14.3% of the total population. The authors concluded that the variability in the measuring and sampling process was due to the variability in defining the population as well as variability in the sources of information (parents, teachers, physicians, etc.). Barkley (1982) suggests that 4% to 5% of school-age children, or about one child in every classroom, are hyperactive. ADHD is also 10 times more common in boys than girls and is more common in families where other members have the disorder.

Assessment

Many children are identified as having ADHD through school based assessment (Atkins & Pelham, 1991). These procedures have typically included a variety of measures including teacher-rating measures, peer rating and sociometric measures, direct observations in classroom and playground settings, and overall academic performance. Atkins and Pelham (1991) stress the importance of using multiple measures to assess the variety of symptoms that occur with this disorder. Characteristics of ADHD include:

1. *Inability to sustain attention.* The most frequently noted characteristic of ADHD is the inability to sustain attention and effort to tasks. Distractibility may be indicated by difficulty in persevering with schoolwork, frequent daydreaming, and overreaction to external events (Cantwell, 1977; Routh, 1980). Shortness of attention span is almost always present in ADHD, and this shortness often persists into adulthood. A child who demonstrates a short attention span typically cannot attend to any academic task for more than a few seconds at a time. As new information is given, the child's attention to the relevant task breaks down and momentarily fixates on something else. The child's thought patterns are too loose and poorly organized to allow enough concentration to finish the task.

2. *Overactivity.* Although distractibility is a primary characteristic of ADHD, overactivity tends to be the most obvious symptom. Overactivity is characterized by intense and undirected energy, fidgetiness, the inability to remain seated, and sometimes a reduced need for sleep (Cantwell, 1977). Children with ADHD may also experience many academic difficulties directly related to the overactivity. Holborrow and Berry (1986) reported that seven times as many children rated as hyperactive were described as having a great deal of difficulty in all academic areas as compared to their nonhyperactive peers.

3. *Impulsivity*. Impulsivity, another characteristic of ADHD, implies a lack of reflection in behavior. Impulsivity may be demonstrated through verbally blurting out and interrupting, physical irritation of others, answering without thinking on educational measures, and a tendency to shift excessively from one activity to another. Impulsive children also tend to use less mature and/or systematic strategies than reflective strategies.

4. *Social skill deficits*. A child who exhibits characteristics of ADHD usually does not fit well into groups. The child is often less mature than most of his or her peers. Outbursts of anger and lack of self-control occur frequently. The child is viewed as immature, irritable, disruptive, demanding, and uncooperative by teachers and peers. These children also have difficulty in establishing and maintaining satisfactory social relationships.

Five hypotheses have been generated regarding the relationship between social skills deficits and children with ADHD: (a) social skills deficits and academic deficits result from the same neurological dysfunction; (b) learning problems prevent the development of social skills; (c) children fail to acquire social skills due to the lack of opportunity in the environment; (d) a dysfunctional family system which causes decreased opportunities for social interaction; and (e) comorbidity where there is a clear overlap between learning disabilities and hyperactivity (Forness & Kavale, 1991).

Prognosis

It was once believed that children's problems with attention, overactivity, impulsivity, and excitability remitted at puberty. However, current research reveals that, although overactivity tends to decrease between the ages of 12 and 16, many of the associated problems persist. Follow-up studies have tracked behavioral difficulties into adolescence and adulthood.

The prognosis for complete remission of all symptoms of hyperactivity is dim. However, many treatment interventions have been used to help individuals with ADHD compensate for many of the deficiencies resulting from the symptoms (Hechtman, Hopkins, Perlman, & Weiss, 1979).

Treatment

A number of interventions have been applied to the characteristics of hyperactivity. These interventions have emanated from several model views including biophysical, behavioral, and cognitive-behavioral.

Biophysical

The biophysical model focuses on the concept of disease. The two types of treatment alternatives which have been typical of this model include pharmacotherapy (drug intervention) and diet-related treatments.

Pharmacotherapy

Stimulant medication has been the most common and most controversial treatment choice for children in the United States (O'Brien & Obrzut, 1986). The medication most often used is methylphenidate (Ritalin®). Other frequently used drugs are Dexedrine® and Cylert®. These three medications are of the class of psychotropic drugs called stimulants. Ritalin® appears to be used about 10 times more frequently than Dexedrine® and Cylert®, usually because its effect on growth is less marked.

Stimulant medication has been effective in reducing overactivity during short periods of time. Barkley (1982) reported that 75% of children with hyperactivity showed a positive response to stimulant therapy. Barkley and Cunningham (1978) reviewed 61 studies relevant to the drug treatment of hyperactivity with stimulants and found that stimulants did change the behaviors and performance of hyperactive children. The greatest effect was on behavioral measures of performance. In contrast, the smallest effects were on academic achievement measures of IQ.

Few studies have evaluated the long-term effects of stimulation medication. The studies which have been conducted have reported no enduring effects of stimulant medication. Children with ADHD who had previously used stimulant medication, but were not medicated at the time of follow-up, did not differ in any way from children who had never received pharmacotherapy.

Many factors may limit the efficacy of the treatment of ADHD with stimulant medication: (a) stimulant medication must be closely prescribed, monitored, and withdrawn under a physician's treatment; (b) long-term studies evaluating stimulant effects have not shown maintenance of desired behaviors over a period of time; (c) stimulant medication is not appropriate for all children with ADHD; and (d) possible side effects of insomnia, anorexia, headache, nausea, moodiness, stomachache, and irritability have been noted with moderate doses of stimulant medication (Barkley, 1981; Gadow, 1986).

In summary, stimulant medication has been shown to have short-term effects in enhancing self-control, interpersonal behavior, and academic performance. However, the possible side effects of stimulant medication, as well as the variability of generalization and maintenance across time and settings, has made this a discouraging treatment choice for many parents and educators.

Dietary Interventions

Dietary and nutritional approaches for controlling hyperactivity are another form of treatment for children with ADHD. These approaches are based on the premise that overactivity is related to the digestion of food substances containing items such as refined sugars and salt compounds. If these products are eliminated from the diet of hyperactive children, it is presumed that overall behavior will improve.

One of the most well-known food plans is the Kaiser Permanente (K-P) diet which was originally described by Feingold (1975). Feingold proposed that the elimination of foods containing artificial colors, flavors, and salicylates (a salt compound found in apples, cherries, oranges, and peaches) could result in the remission of symptoms for 30% to 50% of hyperactive children. Studies have failed to find positive results for dietary control (Connors, 1980; O'Brien & Obrzut, 1986).

Behavioral Interventions

The behavioral model of treatment for ADHD emphasizes the analysis and control of the environment. A fundamental assumption is that all behavior is learned. Behavior modification is very effective in the short term and, in the long term, may be more effective than drug treatment in controlling impulsivity, interpersonal behavior (including self-control skills), and academic performance.

Behavioral treatment programs for the control of hyperactive behaviors typically involve the strengthening and/or weakening of behaviors. This control is accomplished through the delivery of reinforcers and punishers. Reinforcement refers to an increase in the frequency or intensity of the target behavior (Rosenberg, 1985). The praise or rewards used as reinforcers must increase the strength of a target behavior in order to be considered a positive reinforcer. Therefore, it is important to select effective reinforcers that promote the best outcome for increasing behavior. Reinforcers typically used include (a) edibles, (b) praise and attention, (c) performance feedback, (d) tokens, and (e) contingency contracting.

Edibles have been used with a variety of populations. Typical edible reinforcements have included candy, ice cream, and gum.

With research in dietary interventions suggesting that hyperactive behaviors may result from the ingestion of certain foods, the effects of edibles may actually promote hyperactive behaviors. The research here is inconclusive.

Praise and attention are examples of social reinforcers that can be easily administered by parents and teachers in the home and school setting. In order for praise and attention to be effective, delivery should take place immediately after the target behaviors have occurred. The statements of praise should be varied but also be descriptive of the target behavior. For example, instead of saying "good job!" it would be better to say, "you're doing a good job listening to the directions!" It is important for impulsive children to be told exactly about the behaviors for which praise is given.

Performance feedback is defined by Kazdin (1975) as the knowledge of the results of one's efforts toward the attainment of a goal. Studies have shown that feedback is a powerful reinforcer. Charting feedback has shown to be effective in reinforcing the effects of behavioral programming in children with ADHD.

Tokens can take a variety of forms including chips, checkmarks, stickers, or tickets. Tokens can be used to purchase a variety of reinforcers. This process avoids the problem of satiation of reinforcers for children with ADHD. In addition, tokens can be delivered in most situations. Although there are many advantages associated with the use of tokens, one major problem involves record keeping which requires a great deal of instructor time (Axelrod, 1983).

Contingency contracts are written agreements that specify relationships between appropriate child behaviors and the positive consequences to be given. Contingencies in the contract must be the direct result of consultation between the child-parent/teacher dyad. In addition, positive and negative consequences should be specified in advance, making the child responsible for knowledge of all aspects of the contract. Contingency contracts are beneficial for impulsive children because positive and aversive consequences are stated in advance. Consequently, teacher or parental responses to situations cannot be viewed as unfair or arbitrary.

Punishment also has been used to manage the behavior of children with ADHD. Typical punishers have included reprimand, response-cost, and time-out. A *reprimand* is defined as an expression of disapproval directed toward a behavior. Studies of reprimands have shown that, when combined with praise for appropriate behavior, they have been effective in controlling the behavior of children with ADHD (Axelrod, 1983).

Time-out is defined as the contingent removal of the opportunity to earn positive reinforcement (Craighead, 1982). During time-out, a child is placed in a restricted environment following disruptive behavior and remains in isolation for a minimum time period. Return to the classroom is contingent on the passage of the time period in addition to exhibition of appropriate behavior. Many studies have utilized time-out successfully to control problematic classroom behaviors (Drabman, O'Leary, & Spitalnik, 1973).

To achieve maximum benefits with time-out, the child should not have access to reinforcers. Unfortunately, removing all reinforcing events is difficult in a classroom with students having ADHD. Time-out areas may possess many reinforcers. For example, a child may be getting out of work he or she considers to be boring or difficult when put in a time-out situation or setting.

Although behavioral programs have been effective in controlling some behaviors, behavioral procedures alone do not make a hyperactive child more reflective (Kendall & Braswell, 1982; Finch & Spirito, 1980; Messer, 1976). In addition, there is significant evidence showing that behavioral management programs do not generalize across settings or time (Abikoff, 1985; Meichenbaum, 1979). Historically, behavior therapists attempt to change behavior through nonverbal methods, whereas cognitive-behavioral therapists utilize speech as an instrument of change (Abikoff, 1991; Hall, 1980). The combination of traditional behavioral techniques with cognitive training has been shown to be an effective form of treatment for children with ADHD (Kendall & Finch, 1976, 1978).

Cognitive Behavior Modification

Cognitive behavior modification (CBM) is a general category of intervention techniques that attempt to modify behavior and affect by alerting the thought patterns of individuals (Meodor & Ollendick, 1984; Rosenberg, Sindeler, & Stedt, 1985). CBM combines the manipulation of environmental changes with an individual's self-control processes. These processes may include self-instruction, self-monitoring, and/or self-reinforcement (Finch & Spirito, 1980; O'Brien & Obrzut, 1986). CBM interventions place emphasis on self-control. Self-monitoring and self-assessment are strategies frequently used to aid in self-control.

Many researchers have turned to the use of CBM because the effects of traditional operant behavior programs and use of stimulant medication did not generalize across settings or over time (McKinney & Haskins, 1980; Meichenbaum, 1979). CBM interventions are designed to increase self-awareness, self-control, and improve academic behavior (Kendall & Cummings, 1988; Gerber, 1987; Kneedler & Meese, 1988; Loper & Murphy, 1985; Wong, 1985).

CBM with Children with ADHD

Although cognitive-behavioral techniques have been utilized with children who exhibit various handicapping conditions, children with ADHD were among the first groups in which such techniques were implemented. In fact, CBM training procedures have become a popular alternative to pharmacological interventions involving children with ADHD (O'Brien & Obrzut, 1986).

The overall goal of CBM is to develop self-control skills and reflective problem-solving skills, which are both thought to be lacking in children with ADHD. These deficiencies appear to account for difficulties in children's abilities to regulate inattentive, impulsive, and inappropriate interpersonal behaviors. CBM is expected to provide children with the ability to regulate their behavior more appropriately and enhance their social and academic performance (Abikoff, 1991).

Self-talk and modeling are core components of CBM (Lloyd, 1980; Whalen & Henker, 1986). With children involved as active participants in their intervention programs, it is assumed that results will be generalized and maintained with greater frequency and regularity (Meichenbaum & Asarnow, 1979). Although a number of treatment procedures and approaches have been employed, verbal self-instruction and problem-solving training are the most frequently cited as being successful with children with ADHD.

Verbal Self-instruction

Early research by Luria (1961) and Vygotsky (1962) identified the importance of the relationship between internal verbalizations and overt behavior. The assumption of their research was that children assume control over their behavior by internalizing self-directed verbal commands (O'Brien & Obrzut, 1986). From Luria and Vygotsky's work, a theoretical model was proposed in which a child's behavior is first directed by the speech of others, next by the child's own overt speech, and finally by the child's own covert or inner speech.

Meichenbaum and Goodman's (1971) prototypic self-instruction training package was influenced by the work of Luria (1961) and Vygotsky (1962). Their now classic self-instructional package combined modeling, overt and covert rehearsal prompts, feedback and social reinforcement. The program included the following steps:

1. cognitive modeling in which an adult model performed the task while talking aloud and describing cognitive steps to the task;
2. overt external guidance in which the child performed the same task while a model verbalized the instructions to the child;

3. overt self-guidance in which the child performed the task while verbalizing aloud;
4. faded, overt self-guidance in which the child performed the task while instructing him- or herself in a whisper; and
5. covert self-instruction.

Many studies have evaluated the impact of cognitive training (Bornstein & Quevillon, 1976; Cullinan, Epstein, & Silver, 1977; Meichenbaum & Goodman, 1971; Palkes, Freedman, & Stewart, 1972). The results of these studies indicate that verbal self-instruction is effective in increasing reflective problem-solving in children with ADHD. However, maintenance of strategies over a period of time remains questionable.

Another major class of interventions in CBM that also has been shown to be effective with children with ADHD advocates a problem-solving approach to social difficulties. Some versions of self-instructional training have included problem-solving approaches; however, many problem-solving packages do not formally utilize verbal self-instruction.

Problem-solving Interventions

The purpose of problem-solving training is to teach children to generate alternative solutions to interpersonal problems and to evaluate cause-effect relationships. Kneedler (1980) suggested that children exhibiting problems in social skills also have deficiencies in problem-solving skills. In problem-solving situations where there is an uncertainty in response, children with ADHD respond in an impulsive fashion. These children perform less efficiently in social skills than children who perform in a careful, reflective manner (Haskins & McKinney, 1980). Moreover, studies (e.g., Copeland, 1981; Loper, 1980; Hogg, Callias, & Pellegrini,

1986; Meodor & Ollendick, 1984) have indicated that impulsive children utilize less mature strategies than reflective children of the same age. In addition, longitudinal studies have shown that impulsive children evidenced a delayed pattern of strategic development between the ages of 7 and 9, a pattern that seems to be unrelated to intellectual ability (McKinney & Haskins, 1980).

Many studies have identified stages or sequences of problem-solving behavior. D'Zurilla and Goldfried (1971) defined problem-solving as a behavioral process and outlined five stages of problem-solving, including: (a) developing a general orientation to possible problems, (b) developing the ability to identify components of the problem, (c) developing alternative strategies to solve a problem, (d) evaluation of the consequences of the solutions generated, and (e) evaluation of the outcome and self-reinforcement. The authors found in subsequent studies that detailed training in these cognitive operations, each taken individually, led to improvements in problem-solving abilities.

A number of outcome studies have been conducted evaluating the efficacy of problem-solving training programs. In most studies, the problem-solving component involved teaching problem-solving, motor inhibition, attending behavior, and self-direction skills. The procedures included modeling, role-playing, dialogues, and games. Specific objectives included teaching the identification and discrimination of emotions, as well as alternative, consequential, and means-end thinking in application to interpersonal problem-solving. The results of these studies showed overall improvements in all areas of problem-solving ability (Lloyd, 1980; Whalen, Henker, & Hinshaw, 1985).

Problem-solving strategies are important for overcoming self-control deficits. These skills help the child with ADHD to utilize self-control in social situations. The child with ADHD who is able to respond appropriately in social situations is more likely to be accepted by peers and adults.

Social Skills Instruction

Social skills instruction is an approach designed to increase interpersonal skills in critical life situations. Measures of peer acceptance or popularity have been used to define children as socially skilled (Gresham & Elliott, 1987). From a behavioral perspective, social skills are situationally specific behaviors that secure the probability of maintaining positive reinforcement depending on one's social behavior. Social skills also are defined in terms of social validity. In this definition, social skills are defined as those behaviors that predict important social outcomes for children (e.g., peer and teacher acceptance) (Schloss, Schloss, Wood, & Kiehl, 1990). Many impulsive children may know how to interact appropriately with peers and teachers, yet be unable to maintain this skill due to impulsivity in responding (Gresham & Elliott, 1987). For this reason, children with ADHD are appropriate candidates for social skills training.

A recent review by Whalen and Hencker (1991) investigated the social impact of stimulant medication for children with ADHD. They found that children with ADHD have serious and persistent social deficits which cause frequent conflicts in social situations. The children's pragmatic style of social exchange is characterized by deficits in initiating conversation, poor eye contact, and inappropriate conversational behavior. This style is often perceived as being immature, inappropriate, and intrusive. Children with ADHD may exhibit social learning disabilities that hamper their efforts in achieving effective pragmatic skills. Although medication was found to be effective in reducing the disruptive nature of the child's conversational speech, medication did not promote overall social competence. In general, stimulant medication cannot supplement skills that are lacking in children with ADHD. Social skills programs should teach children how to reduce inappropriate social behavior as well as how to establish and build friendships and social relationships.

The Language Impaired ADHD Student

The language impaired ADHD student can be described as displaying age-appropriate articulation skills, average single-word vocabulary, poor communication and social skills, and conversational skills that lack substance (Pate, 1993). A typical assessment profile of this student consists of receptive and/or expressive language delay; poor short-term memory with difficulty following directions; difficulty separating figure ground stimuli; language-based learning problems in academic areas; and limited use of inductive, reflective, and logical thinking (Pate, 1993). Pragmatics are a particular area of difficulty for the student with ADHD. Pragmatic skills are often poor secondary to impulsivity. Students often have difficulty extracting detail and will give information that does not relate to the topic. In addition, students continually change topics, lack appropriate turn-taking skills, and lack the ability to maintain a topic.

Social or behavioral problems are often associated with ADHD. The student may be verbally and physically aggressive, disruptive to others, and easily angered. In addition, attention-seeking behaviors may be accompanied by the tendency to violate rules and blame other people. This student may also seek aggressive solutions to problems. For example, while being teased by a peer, the student with ADHD may choose to physically hurt the person as opposed to solving the problem in a nonviolent manner. Again, all of the above difficulties are secondary to the impulsivity associated with ADHD.

Assessing ADHD Language Abilities

A basic language assessment battery for the student with ADHD should consist of the following: (a) history and data review; (b) two comprehensive language tests (e.g., the Clinical Evaluation of Language Fundamentals-Revised (CELF-R), *Clinical Evalua-*

tion of Language-Preschool [CELF-P], *Test of Language Disorders—Intermediate* [TOLD-I], *Test of Language Disorders—Primary* [TOLD-P], *Woodcock Language Proficiency Battery—Revised* [WLPB-R], *Test of Word Knowledge, Detroit Test of Learning Aptitude* [DTLA], etc.; see Appendix H); (c) normed supplementary probes for language and auditory processing; and (d) descriptive data relative to academic functioning and prosocial skills.

Pate (1993) has outlined some basic behavioral guidelines for completing an assessment: (a) it is important to outline the routine and set clear rules that allow for some flexibility; (b) allow the student choices for where to sit in the testing area; (c) plan breaks in the testing session but allow for activities that can be done in the testing area; (d) be prepared to restrain hands when pointing responses are involved; and (e) have a system prepared to double-score responses. In addition to the above guidelines, Pate (1993) poses four questions to be answered from the assessment data: (a) what age-appropriate skills does the child need? (b) what skills does the child have? (c) what new skill can be acquired through intervention? and (d) what options are available for collaborative support? The answers to these questions lead to the development of a functional, successful intervention plan for the student with ADHD.

Finally, the speech-language evaluation should be part of a multidisciplinary evaluation that assesses all aspects of the student's functions. The multidisciplinary team should include at least a developmental pediatrician, a psychologist, a speech-language pathologist, educators directly involved with the student, and the parents. All members of the team should be familiar with the student. In-depth testing should also evaluate vigilance, sustained attention, focused attention, selected attention, divided attention, and impulsivity. In addition, emotional and/or behavioral problems should be assessed as well as educational performance. Information from the home environment should also be obtained. Many checklists are available for use in both the home and school environment (Child Behavior Checklist,

Conners Parent and Teacher Rating Scales, and Home and School Situations Questionnaires).

Strategies for Curriculum and Classroom-based Language Intervention

Successful intervention in the classroom requires collaborative planning to establish mutual priorities and common goals between the classroom teacher and the speech-language pathologist (SLP). Goals should be selected which include interventions that will have an impact in the classroom. The classroom teacher and the SLP must work together to clarify the procedures, including who will be doing what, when, and where.

The SLP can provide support to the student with ADHD by helping him or her to:

1. Build script knowledge (routines), which is provided to develop verbal and nonverbal socialization strategies through role-playing activities that teach scripts for appropriate communication.
2. Teach strategies to deal with specific classroom experiences, (e.g., test taking, study skills).
3. Teach organizational skills applicable to classroom and homework assignments and unique to the student's learning style.
4. Teach memory strategies.
5. Bombard new vocabulary and functional vocabulary necessary to function in the school environment.
6. Teach self-evaluation and pro-social skills. (Pate, 1993)
7. Adjust expectations of the student.

The whole language approach has recently emerged as an effective tool with children with ADHD. The SLP should provide classroom-based services which focus on interventions specific to the curriculum. Some specific suggestions for curriculum-based language intervention are:

1. Provide naturalistic intervention in the classroom.
2. Develop script building.
3. Use semantic word mapping.
4. Use the Shared Book Experience.
5. Use a Dialogue Journal.
6. Introduce prereading and prewriting activities.
7. Use outlining and flow charting to aid in study skills and note taking. (Pate, 1993)

Finally, as the child with ADHD is included in the general education classroom, teachers may need to modify programs for the student. The following are some educational recommendations for use with the student with ADHD who has language deficits:

1. Be sure that rules and schedules are clear by posting pictures of list of rules and reviewing rules regularly.
2. Organize ideas. Introduce outlining, highlighting, and mind-maps in early grades.
3. Develop problem-solving skills. Practice brainstorming to make decisions and model good problem-solving strategies aloud.
4. Limit distractions in the classroom. Surround the student with calm, well-focused students; avoid focused seat work if a group activity is in progress; and use earphones without sound to screen out noise.

5. Engage the child in activities. Use cooperative learning activities; use peer tutors alternating helper-learner roles; teach the child verbal self-instruction to talk through activities; and avoid lengthy assignments that involve copying or worksheet activities.
6. Give self-paced rather than timed tests.
7. Give simple directions or record the instructions for the student on a tape to be used on a Walkman®, which can then be used at home and school.
8. Adjust teacher and parent expectations of the child in various situations.
9. Beware of negative reinforcement.
10. Provide a setting where the child is allowed to move around without being penalized.

Summary

ADHD is one of the most common disorders diagnosed in the pediatric population. Children do not outgrow ADHD; many of the problems of attention, distractibility, overarousal, impulsivity, and difficulty delaying gratification persist into adulthood. The age at which most referrals occur is when the child first enters an organized classroom setting. Typically, problems in the areas of behavior, social, cognition, academics, emotional and physical deficits may coexist with the ADHD. Although there are no diagnostic assessments specific to this population, there are reliable evaluations which can be used to support or refute the deficit. Speech and language testing is one component of a multidisciplinary evaluation used to diagnose associated deficits to ADHD. Interventions should be individualized to the student's learning profile and style with emphasis on classroom curriculum-based consultation. As an SLP working with the child with ADHD, it is important to be familiar with the many cognitive and behavioral interventions to enhance language intervention. Equally important is the role of the SLP in collaborating with the classroom teacher in designing the most effective and functional program for the student to be successful in the school setting.

CHAPTER 3

Tourette Syndrome

Definition

Tourette syndrome is the most severe of the neurological disorders known collectively as tic disorders. Tic disorders represent a clinical spectrum ranging from the mild transient tic to the more severe, Tourette syndrome (TS) (Singer & Walkup, 1991).

Tics are the most common involuntary movement disorder of childhood. According to Torup (1972), between 4% and 23% will experience tics during their lives. Tics are defined as involuntary, rapid, and repetitive movements that occur suddenly and irregularly. *Tics* often involve muscle groups of the face, neck, shoulders, and arms. Tic disorders occur along a continuum ranging from a mild transitory condition to a complex, persistent set of behaviors that may be disabling to the individual (Roddy, 1989). Disorders involving tics are generally divided into categories according to age of onset, duration of symptoms, and the presence of vocal or phonic tics in addition to motor tics (Bruun, Cohen, & Leckman, 1990).

The first type of tic disorder is known as transient tic disorder. By definition, these are common tics that involve 1 muscle group and last less than 1 year. These tics may include eye blinking, nose puckering, grimacing, and squinting (Bruun, Cohen, & Leckman, 1990; Colligan, 1989; Lehrer, 1987). Although less common, transient vocalizations may include various throat sounds, humming, or other noises. Transient tics often begin during the school years (between ages 5 and 15), and the prognosis for spontaneous remission is good with no medical or psychological treatment necessary (Golden & Hood, 1982). Transient tics are most noticeable with excitement or fatigue (Bruun, Cohen, & Leckman, 1990). If the tics last longer than a year and are accompanied by attentional, learning, or behavioral problems, the child should be referred for a complete multidisciplinary assessment including a medical evaluation.

Chronic tic disorders differ from transient tic disorders in the duration of the tics (usually over many years) and in the unchanging nature of the tics. Chronic tics may persist in the same state for years.

Chronic multiple (motor or phonic) tic disorders are defined by the presence of tics for more than 12 months. The tics usually are either motoric or vocalic in form (Singer & Walkup, 1991).

Tourette syndrome (Gilles de la Tourette syndrome) is the most severe of the continuum of tic disorders. It is a chronic, debilitating tic disorder characterized by both motor and phonic tics. According to DSM-IV (APA, 1994), the diagnostic criteria for Tourette's disorder include:

> (a) both multiple motor and one or more vocal tics have been present at some time during the illness, although not necessarily concurrently; (b) the tics occur many times a day (usually in bouts) nearly every day or intermittently throughout a period of more than one year, and during this period there was never a tic-free period of more than three consecutive months; (c) the disturbance causes marked distress or significant impairment in social, occupational, or other important areas of functioning; (d) the onset age is before 18 years; and (e) the disturbance is not due to direct physiological effects of a substance (e.g. stimulants) or a general medical condition (e.g. Huntington's disease or postviral encephalitis). (p. 103)

Several researchers have pointed out that the APA definition does not adequately portray the range of behavioral problems that are commonly associated with TS including academic problems, attentional problems and obsessive-compulsive behavior (Bruun, Cohen, & Leckman, 1990; Singer & Walkup, 1991).

Characteristics of Children with Tourette Syndrome

Motor Tics

Motor tics can take a variety of forms from simple to complex. Simple tics involve a limited number of muscle groups and include: eye blinking, mouth opening, facial grimacing, head jerking, nose twitching, shoulder shrugging, tongue protrusion, arm or leg jerking, lip licking, and body jerking. Complex motor tics, on the other hand, involve several muscle groups. Only 10% of persons diagnosed with Tourette syndrome exhibit the complex motor tic of copropraxia, which consists of socially unacceptable, obscene gestures (Roddy, 1989). Complex motor tics include jumping, finger snapping, hitting self or others, wiping of face, touching self or others, kicking, smelling hands or objects, twiddling of hair, skipping, and copropraxia.

Vocal Tics

Vocal tics vary in individuals diagnosed with TS. These tics include a continuum from noises produced in the throat to the shouting of syllables, words, and phrases. Vocal tics include throat clearing, barking, grunting, snorting, squealing, stammering, sniffing, stuttering, coughing, hissing, screaming, noisy breathing, humming, groaning, echolalia, palilalia, and coprolalia. The latter three types of vocal tics are less common. Echolalia involves the repetition of the last word or phrase of another person. Palilalia includes the repetition of one's own last word or phrase. Coprolalia involves the use of obscenities. Coprolalia, once thought to be a distinguishing characteristic of TS, actually occurs in only 10% of the population diagnosed with TS.

The symptoms of TS can be diagnosed as mild, moderate, or severe, based on their complexity and the degree to which they impair or disrupt the child's daily activities. There also may be a great deal of variability in the frequency, symptomatology, and severity over time. Tics tend to wax and wane. The tics may become worse during periods of stress or improve when the child is involved in something enjoyable (Bruun, Cohen, & Leckman, 1990; Roddy, 1989).

An important point about tics is that they are involuntary. Drawing attention to the tics may actually cause an increase in the frequency with which they occur. The child can make a conscious effort to suppress a tic temporarily and be successful. However, this suppression creates a build up of stress that the child must release.

Tics also can change over a period of time. New tics may develop as old ones disappear. Tics do not only occur during the daytime. Sleep studies have shown that motor and vocal tics can occur during all stages of sleep. Children with TS may also have other sleep disturbances including an increased number of awakenings and enuresis (Glaze, Frost, & Jankovic, 1983).

Tourette syndrome and some of the associated problems are reported to be of genetic origin. Several family members may exhibit one or more of the motor tics associated with the syndrome. However, TS may go undiagnosed for years if family members are unaware that this genetic syndrome exists in their lineage. Family members often experience feelings of guilt about having transmitted these problems to their child. For this reason, it is important to be sensitive in questioning parents about the nature of their child's problems (Bronheim, 1991).

Incidence

Although Gilles de la Tourette syndrome is uncommon, it is probably underdiagnosed. Bruun (1984) estimated that its prevalence in the United States is about 0.05%. He further reported that males are affected about three times as frequently as females, and all racial groups are represented in the figure. However, studies in the United States revealed a large number of cases in Ashkenazi Jews (Eldridge, Sweet, Shapiro, & Arena, 1975).

Associated Disorders

Attention Deficit Hyperactivity Disorder (ADHD), Obsessive Compulsive Disorder (OCD), learning disabilities, and behavioral disorders are all associated with Tourette syndrome.

Attention Deficit Hyperactivity Disorder

As many as 50 to 60% of children with TS are also diagnosed as ADHD, much higher than the general population. The incidence is 6 to 10 times higher in males and 20 to 40 times higher in females (Matthews, 1988). Short attention spans, concentration difficulties, distractibility, impulsivity, and hyperactivity have been documented in TS (Bruun, Cohen & Leckman, 1990; Singer & Walkup, 1991). The attentional difficulties have been documented to precede the onset of symptoms of TS and may worsen as the tics develop. In addition, children often are referred for the symptoms of ADHD rather than the tics prior to the diagnosis of TS. Several studies have reported that the majority of patients with TS present first with the characteristics of ADHD, with the development of motor and vocal tics occurring an average of 2.4 years later (Comings & Comings, 1987). In addition, siblings of children with TS were often diagnosed with ADHD. Comings (1990) reported that children with TS and ADHD have more problems in behavior and conduct than children with pure ADHD. In general, it has been reported in many cases that the more severe the TS, the more pronounced the ADHD will be. Fidgetiness and overactivity in the classroom may be directly related to either the motor tic activity or the hyperactivity (Matthews, 1988). External and internal distractions may disrupt the child's ability to remain on task or carry out instructions for the task's completion. In terms of impact, the ADHD has been found to have a more adverse effect on functioning than the tic symptoms. At times, the tics may require no intervention, whereas the ADHD deficits may require intense intervention (Matthews, 1988). Issues related to intervention will be discussed later in this chapter.

Obsessive Compulsive Disorder

Obsessive-compulsive disorder (OCD) is also present in children diagnosed with TS. Characteristics of OCD include the presence of recurrent behaviors and/or thoughts that intrude on the consciousness. These usually are involuntary and distressing to the child. The characteristics can become debilitating when they cause significant impairment. Compulsions consist of the behaviors carried out in response to the obsessions. Possible compulsive behaviors include repeated hand washing, rituals of counting, and cleaning things or checking things frequently (door locks, windows, etc.). Obsessive symptoms may include fears of contamination with dirt or germs, fears of loved ones being harmed, and other thoughts or images that intrude on consciousness (Singer & Walkup, 1991).

Singer and Walkup (1991) noted that an overlap is observed among compulsive behaviors, complex tics, and obsessive thoughts. Their example was that a recurring desire to touch an object or part of the body may be either a complex motor tic or a compulsive behavior. Like tics, OCD symptoms come and go. They arise when there is stress, and are also unable to be controlled.

Learning Disabilities

Learning disabilities are another deficit associated with TS. Studies have shown that 50% of children diagnosed with TS also have concomitant learning disabilities (Burd, Kerbeshian, Cook, Bornhoeff, & Fisher, 1988; Golden, 1984; Hagin, Beecher, Pagano, & Kreeger, 1982; Hagin & Kugler, 1988). These studies used assessments evaluating the relationship between IQ and academic achievement as the method for identification of the learning disabilities. A more recent study on prevalence rates showed that, in a rural population of clinically treated children with TS, 51% evidenced a learning disability in at least one subject and 21% exhibited a learning disability in two or more subject areas (Burd, Kauffman, & Kerbeshian, 1992). The results of this study suggest that children diagnosed with TS need to be evaluated continuously for a learning disability. The need for evaluation is substantiated regardless of the age of onset or the diagnosis of the TS.

Once the tics are brought under control with medication, the school problems often become the focus of attention. The learning disabilities associated with TS usually are manifested in the areas of written language, arithmetic, and reading. A large number of children with TS also have visual-motor integration problems (Bronheim, 1991; Matthews, 1988). Tasks that require children to see the material, process the information, and write it down are difficult. Lengthy assignments often produce frustration, particularly when there is a time limit. Legibility of written work is also often poor. Many children with TS have organizational problems, which may contribute to their written language difficulties. For example, writing a story involves more than a motor task. The process includes planning the story, preparing a title and an outline of events, and developing a theme. Children with organizational problems will have difficulty with the task of planning and executing these written language activities.

Some children with TS have difficulties that affect language. There are two types: language-based learning deficits and language problems that are specific to the tics of TS (Bronheim, 1991). Certainly, any of the written language problems previously described can be language-based. Such organizational problems also can interfere with auditory processing, semantics, syntax, and pragmatics. Particularly problematic for children with TS is the area of pragmatics. Tics have a tendency to interfere with language expression as opposed to comprehension. Children with TS often stutter, have trouble relating stories and information, demonstrate word-finding difficulties, and use loud or "pressured" speech.

Interpersonal communication also can be affected if the tics are expressed rather than suppressed. If words are repeated, as in echolalia, or if the tics are explosive, the listener may become easily distracted and disengaged in the conversation. In addition, the situation may deteriorate further if the child with TS has additional attention problems and is unable to maintain an effective conversation. These types of deficits can lead to increased pragmatic and socialization problems.

Another problematic academic area for children with TS is arithmetic. Many studies have shown that children with TS perform significantly below age expectations on tests involving rote learning and computation due to difficulties with attention and graphomotor abilities (Matthews, 1988). These children often do better on oral arithmetic word problems and are capable of applying mathematical concepts to real-life situations (Matthews, 1988).

Many parents of children with TS report that their children have difficulties in learning to read. Comings and Comings (1987) reported that 27% of patients with TS have some problems with dyslexia and 41% have poor retention of material that was read. Recent studies of dyslexia suggest that the individual's sensory input is normal, but the proper storage of images of words in the memory is defective. Therefore, words are stored without a complete set of phonetic clues. When a child with dyslexia needs to recall a word, he or she frequently cannot do so because not enough clues have been retained (Comings, 1990).

An additional problem is that some children suffer from blocking. They cannot read quickly because they get stuck on sentences or words. The compulsive need to start again at the beginning, repeat a word, count words in a sentence, and so on can interfere with the ability to retain and process information that was read (Comings & Comings, 1987).

In summary, children with TS often have significant learning problems throughout their school years, including difficulties with reading, written language, pragmatics, mathematics, and visual and auditory perception problems. More research is needed in all of these areas to document the specific deficits that are characteristic to children with TS.

Behavioral Disorders

Conduct disorder occurs in many children with TS. Several types of behavior problems have been identified, including aggressiveness, lying, stealing, starting fires, vandalism, and fighting. Behavior problems may in part be a response to having a stigmatizing disorder, may be due to the accompanying diagnosis of ADHD, or may not be attributable to the tics at all. In terms of treatment, studies have shown that the behaviors seem to be resistant to psychotherapy and medication (Singer & Walkup, 1991; Steff, 1984).

Assessment

Clinical Assessment

The diagnosis of TS must be based on an accurate history from the parents. The nature, severity, frequency, and degree of disruption produced by the motor and vocal tics need to be carefully assessed from the time of their emergence to the present. Information also should be obtained from the family regarding the interference of the tics with the child's experiences at home, during school, and in the community (Bruun, Cohen, & Leckman, 1990).

During the course of the evaluation, family issues, including feelings of guilt, need to be assessed. Parents need to be educated and informed about the etiology and treatment for the disorder. In addition, information should be obtained regarding the child's school performance and functioning.

A neurological examination should be included as part of the clinical assessment. This examination should document any soft signs which suggest disturbances in the body scheme and integration of motor control. Additional studies may include: (a) an EEG and/or CAT scan; (b) serum electrolytes, calcium, phosphorous, copper, ceruloplasmin, and liver function tests; (c) a behavioral pedigree of the extended family; and (d) a review of the history of previous medications. The final study may be particularly important if the child is already on stimulant medication to determine the positive and negative effects of various medications (Bruun, Cohen, & Leckman, 1990).

Frequently, TS is not diagnosed appropriately. Comings and Comings (1987) documented three major factors for missed diagnosis: (a) lack of familiarity with the syndrome; (b) suppressibility of the motor and vocal tics for several hours; and (c) the belief that coprolalia must be present.

For these reasons, it is important that an educational assessment be performed to document any deficits related to attentional, learning, or behavioral problems. In many cases, the child with TS may first be diagnosed with ADHD and/or learning disabilities. If this is the case, it is important for school personnel and specialists to be aware of the presenting symptoms of TS so that a proper diagnosis is not missed.

Educational Assessment

School is a problem for many children with TS. Motor tics can cause three types of problems. The tics may interfere with reading and/or writing. Rapid eye-blinking makes it difficult for the child to keep his or her eyes on the page. The tics also may become a source of social ridicule by the child's peers. Finally, teachers may misinterpret the tics as deliberate misbehavior and discipline the child for something that cannot be controlled (Comings, 1990).

Children with TS should be monitored even if they do not show any particular academic, social, or emotional difficulties at the time of diagnosis. If problems are occurring at home or in school, an in-depth evaluation is warranted. This evaluation should be conducted by a multidisciplinary team consisting of the child's parents, physician, and classroom teacher, as well as the school's principal, special education teacher(s), nurse, psychologist, speech-language pathologist, and social worker.

All areas of academics should be assessed including reading, writing, speaking, listening, pragmatics, mathematics, spelling, and handwriting skills. Attentional deficits may be assessed through direct observation and/or the use of parent/teacher checklists. The team also needs to evaluate how the child is accepting the disorder emotionally and how TS has affected his self image. As always, it is important to obtain a developmental and educational history from the parents. This type of evaluation does not differ from most in-depth evaluations for learning disabilities except that the learning problems are secondary to the TS.

Once the evaluation is completed, the team then can make a determination for the best type of educational placement for the child, a self-contained classroom or integration in the regular classroom with support services from special education teachers and SLPs. Placement decisions for the child with TS should consider all of the child's needs including academic, social, and emotional domains.

Treatment

Treatment for the child with TS includes treatment for the tics, which is pharmacological, and interventions for the secondary characteristics that affect school performance.

Pharmacological Treatment

Pharmacological treatment for tic disorders is based on symptomology. There is no cure for TS. The decision to use drugs depends on the severity of the tics and whether they interfere with normal development (Singer & Walkup, 1991). In some cases, when a child is diagnosed with TS, drug treatment may not be indicated if the child is not having problems with academics, social interactions, or self-image. Many times, the associated problems of ADHD, OCD, or behavioral problems present a greater deficit. Selection of the correct medication depends on defining the target symptoms. For example, children with ADHD or OCD in addition to TS may not respond to medications that suppress motor or vocal tics (Singer & Walkup, 1991).

Three medications have been shown to be effective in controlling tics: (a) haloperidol (Haldol®); (b) clonidine (Catapres®), and pimozide (Orap®). As with all medications, the dosage should be monitored and adjusted to the child's condition at a particular time and to determine whether continued use of the medication is warranted (Roddy, 1989; Singer & Walkup, 1991).

Haloperidol is the medication chosen most frequently for treatment. It has been shown to be effective in treating 80% of the cases. Unfortunately, there are frequent side-effects associated with even the lowest dosage (< 1 mg). These side effects include: (a) excessive fatigue, (b) euphoria, (c) weight gain, (d) depression, (e) school phobias, (f) anxiety, (g) movement abnormalities, and (h) agitation (Singer & Walkup, 1991).

Clonidine reduces tics in some children although it has not been shown to be as effective as haloperidol. In addition, some children have shown improvement in attention and OCD problems when using this treatment. The effects of this medication occur slowly. The effectiveness of this treatment in reducing the tics may not be evident for up to 3 months. The most notable side effect of clonidine is sedation. In addition, if the medication is abruptly withdrawn, the tics may intensify.

Pimozide is a more recently approved drug that has also been shown to be effective in reducing tics. In some studies, pimozide has been shown to have fewer side effects than haloperidol (Singer & Walkup, 1991). However, other studies have reported that this drug causes electrocardiogram changes in some patients. Therefore, if this drug is chosen for treatment, the patient should be monitored by ECG (Roddy, 1989).

The use of stimulants to treat the child with both TS and ADHD is a difficult treatment decision. The most common stimulant used to treat ADHD is methylphenidate, better known as Ritalin®. This drug may increase tics in some children. Obviously, if the tics increase in severity, the use of stimulant medication should be discontinued. However, for many children, the symptoms caused by the ADHD are more disabling than the tics. In these instances, behavioral and educational approaches should be considered first to control the ADHD. These approaches include behavior management, cognitive behavior management, proper school placement, and others. When these approaches are not effective in reducing the ADHD, trial dosages of one of the three pharmacological treatments are recommended. If the child improves overall and the tics do not worsen, the medication is continued. However, if the ADHD improves, but the tics worsen, the medication is discontinued and another stimulant is recommended for a trial period (Singer & Walkup, 1991).

Educational Intervention

Many children with TS show great improvement in the reduction of vocal and motor tics during the mid-teenage years. Unfortunately, the associated learning and behavioral problems may continue. However, with proper educational intervention throughout their school years, children may learn to cope with and accommodate to their symptoms. The key is proper intervention for both the child with TS and his or her parents and everyone who is involved in the education of this child. Because the child's associated deficits may involve language-based learning disabilities, the SLP must monitor the child and consult with his or her teachers frequently to be sure that no problems are emerging.

The SLP who is knowledgeable about the child with TS should be involved from the beginning of assessment. Even if direct speech-language therapy services are not warranted at the time, the SLP should maintain regular contact with the child's teachers to provide guidance regarding activities involving all areas of language (written language, pragmatics, word-retrieval, etc.). If the child is identified as having language-based learning deficits, the SLP should address the areas of need. With the recent adoption of inclusion, it is likely that the child with TS will be integrated in the regular classroom unless his or her behavioral problems are too intense. If this is the case, collaborative consultation may be the method of service delivery. The areas of intervention, of course, are individualized for each child; however, pragmatics and written language skills have been identified continuously as areas of need. Certainly, the use of the whole language approach would be an effective means of integrating all areas of language, including reading, writing, speaking, listening, and processing. In addition, scaffolding may be used with the whole language approach and has been shown to be an effective way to increase pragmatic competence. Direct social skills training may also be indicated to increase interpersonal communication skills.

The SLP also may provide the link between the school-based personnel and the parents of the child with TS. In many cases, the school will not have a wealth of information regarding the educational, behavioral, and emotional needs of children with TS and their families. In this role, the SLP is responsible for educating all school personnel involved with the student regarding TS and his or her possible educational needs. The following are some guidelines suggested for the management of school problems that also may be used to educate school personnel.

1. Obtain proper diagnosis: Many children struggle through years of problems because of missed or incorrect diagnoses. The associated symptoms of ADHD or OCD may be the primary diagnosis when the primary diagnosis is really TS.

2. Provide one-to-one help through the school system, if possible, or obtain a tutor to provide the extra attention that is needed.

3. For tic symptoms, give the child frequent breaks from the classroom to relieve the tics. In addition, provide an area where the child may go to release the tics, such as the nurse's office or resource room. Educate other students who are in contact with the child with TS so that they are more sensitive to his or her feelings.

4. To control ADHD problems, provide the appropriate medical and school treatment as needed. As for other children with ADHD, it is important to provide structure in the school day. Other suggestions are: (a) allow freedom for movement within the classroom, (b) change tasks frequently, (c) break down assignments, (d) help the child to organize long-range projects by establishing shorter time frames when things are due, (e) help the child to organize notebooks and folders so the student can be more organized with homework and schoolwork, (f) implement an appropriate behavior modification system, and (g) reduce the length of homework assignments.

5. Allow for modifications in testing (which should be documented in the Individualized Education Plan). Allow tests without time restrictions as much as possible. In testing formats, children with TS have difficulty with space. Suggestions may include having each problem or question isolated on a section of the student's paper or allowing the student to use an index card that has a window cut out so only one question can be read at a time.

6. For visual motor integration, auditory processing, and fine motor skill deficits: (a) allow the use of a word processor, (b) recommend occupational therapy, (c) do not penalize the child for spelling errors or poor handwriting, (d) give clear, simple directions, (e) present material in both auditory and visual modes, (f) allow reports to be given orally, (g) have a

peer act as a note taker or allow the use of a tape recorder, and (h) allow the student a place to go where he or she can repeat the directions to him or herself without disturbing others.

7. Educate parents, school personnel, peers, and anyone who is in contact with the child with TS. The education provided will alleviate many of the misunderstandings about TS and allow for acceptance of the child (Comings & Comings, 1987; Connors, 1990; Favish, 1990).

Summary

Tourette syndrome is a neurological disorder that is the most severe of the classification of tic disorders. Motoric and verbal tics are common to children with TS, although they may not be the most disabling characteristics of TS. The associated deficits of attention deficit hyperactivity disorder, learning disabilities, obsessive compulsive disorder, and behavioral problems may interfere more with the child's functioning in the home, school, and community than the presence of tics.

Children with TS often are first diagnosed with one of the associated disorders during their early school years. For this reason, speech-language pathologists must be knowlegeable about TS, its associated deficits, assessment, and treatment. It is clear that much more research needs to be conducted in the area of the types of learning disabilities that are present in this population. Some of the literature has supported the existence of language-based learning disabilities in TS. Therefore, the SLP should be a part of the multidisciplinary team to rule out these deficits. At the very least, the SLP should be able to provide education to school personnel, the child's peers, and parents so that those involved with the child can understand that the symptoms, mainly the tics, are involuntary, and are only one defining quality of this child (see Appendix C). This acceptance will help in effectively integrating the child with TS in the school setting most appropriate for his or her needs, whether it is a regular or a special needs classroom.

CHAPTER 4

Children with Fragile X Syndrome

Definition

Fragile X is a genetic disorder that leads to a constellation of some or many of the following: known physical characteristics and anomalies, mental retardation, learning disabilities, and dysfunction of sensory integration. Fragile X can co-occur with autism and pervasive developmental disorder (Scharfenaker, 1990). Clinicians may have individuals with fragile X on existing caseloads before the genetic basis of their disorders is diagnosed.

Incidence

Fragile X, or fra(X), is one of the most common sources of mental retardation in males, but accounts for only about 7% of retardation in females. The level of retardation associated with fra(X) also tends to be milder in females. It is *the* most common inherited cause for retardation. Incidence estimates vary, but it appears that about 1 in 1000 males born have fragile X, and about 1 in 2000 females have the genetic condition (Scharfenaker, 1990). However, there has been no sampling of the population at large so it is not yet known with certainty how often it occurs.

Not all people showing expression of the fra(X) gene have mental retardation, and the likelihood that an individual does *not* have retardation is increased if the person is female. But even some boys with the disorder have intelligence within the normal range along with learning disabilities and/or behavior problems. Approximately 1 in 750 females born is a carrier of the fragile X gene, and she may or may not show expression of the disordered gene. About half of all female *carriers* will show the fra(X) gene on chromosomal testing. Those who do not will usually be unaffected. A carrier will, however, pass on the gene in a predictable pattern. There are also occasionally male carriers of the fra(X) gene, that is, men who show no expression of fra(X) traits but who can pass the gene on to their daughters (only daughters receive an X chromosome from fathers).

Importance for Professionals

A good deal is known about possible speech and language and other disorders a child, especially a male, with fragile X is likely to have. For that reason, it is important for SLPs and other professionals to know about fra(X) and its implications for a child's development and learning as well as likely strengths and weaknesses. Because of the ubiquity of this genetic condition, its increasing severity as it passes through generations, and the variability of its expression, experts recommend that any person presenting with mental retardation, learning disabilities, or "autistic-like" characteristics should be considered a candidate for genetic testing for possible fra(X) condition. Further, anyone presenting with at least one of the physical and behavioral features along with mental retardation or learning disabilities should definitely be referred to a genetics specialist for testing (Scharfenaker, 1990). These guidelines are important because, although diagnosis has been increasing, it is still a relatively newly described condition. Therefore, its existence in a particular child is not always diagnosed as early as it could be.

The Genetic Underpinnings

Fragile X syndrome was originally called Martin-Bell syndrome after the researchers who were among the earliest to describe the existence of X-linked mental retardation in families. An X chromosome with what looks like a broken tip on the bottom end of the long arm of the X chromosome was first identified by Lubs (1969) (see Figure 4–1). Recall that chromosomes are the structures, ordinarily occurring in 23 pairs, in each cell in the body. Each chromosome is composed of a long series of genes. Within the genes is the information dictating the characteristics of the person.

Knowledge of the fragile X syndrome was not often applied to specific cases during the 1970s. In the 1980s, the number of individuals receiving the diagnosis began to balloon. Some older children, adolescents, and adults diagnosed with mental retardation, but for whom no source was known, finally had a source for the retardation and other impairments. In 1991, the fragile X gene on the X chromosome was discovered. Researchers do not yet know what the gene ordinarily does when its normal form has not been disrupted. This information eventually will allow

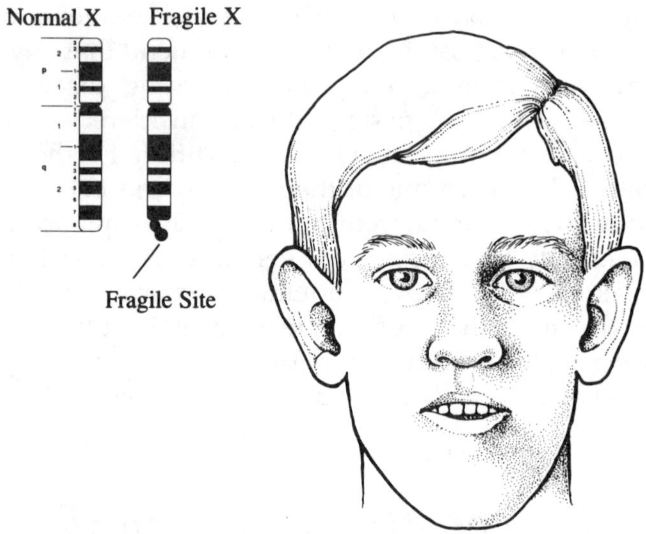

Figure 4–1

An adolescent with fragile X syndrome has an unusual, elongated face, large ears, and a prominent jaw. He usually develops enlarged testicles. Younger children have more subtle facial alterations. The fragile X chromosome is shown, with the terminal pinched off portion.

them to design a treatment for fra(X). Discovery of the gene involved in fragile X led to the ability to identify carriers more accurately as well as the design of a prenatal test from amniocentesis (McConkie-Rosell, 1991). Before this discovery, accurate genetic testing for the disordered gene was more difficult and worsened with age. That was because there is wide variability in expression of the gene in various cells within the body of either a person expressing the syndrome or in a carrier. It also happens that, as a person ages, fewer and fewer cells show the disordered gene. Therefore, in a person showing no clinical expression of fra(X), it was difficult to determine possible carrier status.

In an inherited genetic defect such as fra(X), the underlying problem is present in the genetic material passed to the embryo.

In X-linked genetic disorders, the contributing parent usually is the mother. She may or may not show any clinical expression of the syndrome herself. Boys typically are more affected by the fra(X) syndrome than girls because they only have one X chromosome: the defective one. That X, of course, always comes from the mother, whereas the child's Y chromosome comes from his father. In girls, the existence of the same site on the unaffected X chromosome somehow ameliorates some or all of the effects of the defective gene. Unlike most X-linked disorders, some males showing no clinical expression of fra(X) have been found to be carriers. These carriers pass the defective gene on to daughters who themselves do not show clinical nor genetic evidence of the disorder. The daughters continue the chain by being at risk for having fra(X) disordered children. Research has shown that the syndrome is expressed in progressively stronger fashion and more frequently in successive generations. In fra(X) the identified gene causing all the clinical characteristics that can be seen is designated as fMR-1 (McConkie-Rosell, 1991).

Characteristics of Children with Fragile X

Physical Characteristics

Some of the characteristics described here either apply only to males with fra(X) or are usually seen only in males. In some other cases, the characteristic can be present in females with fra(X) but may be less strongly expressed. The characteristics discussed are those most commonly observed in individuals diagnosed with fra(X) (Chudley & Hagerman, 1987). A person with the genetic disorder may have many of these characteristics or very few because of the variability in expression of the fra(X) gene (Table 4–1).

Boys with the syndrome often are macrocephalic with protruding ears and a prominent forehead. The palatal shape is a high arch, with an increased risk for cleft palate, and there is a nar-

Table 4–1. Possible effects of the Fragile X syndrome.

Ability	Possible Effects
Physical	Long, narrow face Prominent ears Macroorchidism Hyperextensible joints High palate Seizures Vision problems Prognathism Mitral valve prolapse
Sensory and motor integration	Hypotonia Dyspraxia Difficulty with transitions and changes Abnormal sensitivity in various sensory systems Hypersensitivity to eye contact Poor awareness of body in space
Cognitive	Mental retardation Learning disabilities Good imitation skills
Speech and language	Delayed and disordered speech and language Impaired receptive language processing Poor intelligibility Rapid rate Cluttering Difficulty staying on topic Echolalia and/or perseveration Vocabulary strength Poor comprehension and use of communicative gestures Receptive language better than expressive language

(continued)

Table 4–1. *continued*

Ability	Possible Effects
Social	High social anxiety Good sense of humor Impaired social interaction

Note: Not all children with fra(X) will have all of these characteristics.

row, flat nasal bridge. Boys may have epicanthal folds at their eyes, ptosis, simian palmar creases, pectus excavatum, and flat feet. There is usually hypotonia throughout the body with hyperextensible joints. If the boys do not present with a long, narrow face before puberty, they often will *after* puberty's effects on growth. Along with puberty also usually comes macroorchidism (large testicles), prognathism, and frequently mitral valve prolapse. The flat feet, pectus excavatum, high arched palate, and possibly the mitral valve prolapse, are thought to be the result of connective tissue dysplasia during fetal development. Individuals with fra(X) are more prone to hernias and dislocated joints because of the loose condition of connective tissue throughout the body. Physical characteristics that occur more rarely include scoliosis and abnormalities such as club foot (Hagerman, 1992) (see Table 4–1).

Girls with the syndrome often show fewer and less severely expressed characteristics. They may have the hyperextensible joints and the head and facial characteristics of fra(X) (i.e., the long face, slightly prominent ears, prominent forehead). In girls the physical characteristics sometimes occur in the absence of learning or behavior disorders.

It is common to see hyperextensible finger joints listed as one of the characteristics defining fra(X) (Scharfenaker, 1990). Actually, many of the children have loose, or lax, joints *throughout* their bodies. Joint laxity is part of the disrupted development of connective tissue for which the fragile X gene is responsible. This loose connection at the joints is, in part, one of the underlying reasons children with fra(X) often experience delayed motor development. It is also a reason why, even when a motor skill is attained, the quality of the movement or the stability of one muscle group for movement in another may be poorer.

Another very common characteristic associated with the fragile X gene is generalized hypotonia. Low muscle tone combines with joint laxity in affecting the rate of acquisition and quality of gross and fine motor abilities. It is evident in infancy and is a condition which the child will work to overcome throughout life.

Boys with fra(X) are also at a greater than usual risk for recurring otitis media. The first episode often occurs before 6 months of age. It is not yet clear whether this is another manifestation of connective tissue dysplasia or of the different shapes of head and facial characteristics. Regardless, these children often need PE tubes at an early age to avoid hearing loss. Awareness of the increased risk for otitis media is another reason that early diagnosis of fra(X) is so important.

Fra(X) also carries a higher than normal risk of vision problems. The most common disorder is strabismus, but near- or farsightedness, and nystagmus abnormalities are also more common than usual (Hagerman, 1992). For this reason, again a need for early diagnosis, the child's vision should be evaluated as early as possible.

Some abnormalities in brain anatomy or physiology have been associated with a fra(X) diagnosis. About 20% of the children with this diagnosis also have a seizure disorder with variability in the types of seizures noted. Ventricles in the brain also have been found to be enlarged in at least some individuals with fra(X), and a part of the cerebellum (the posterior cerebellar vermis) has been found to be smaller (Hagerman, 1992).

The inability to process incoming information in a normal way is a hallmark feature of fragile X and occurs in many individuals, both boys and girls, with the disorder. Two overlapping clusters of characteristics are the result of inaccurate information processing: sensory integration dysfunction and attention deficit disorder with or without hyperactivity. A person with fra(X) may present with one or both of these clusters of characteristics (Scharfenaker, 1990). Attention deficit disorder and hyperactivity associated with fra(X) will be discussed fully in the section on attention and activity level. Sensory integration dysfunction is discussed in the next section.

Sensory Integration

In the theory of sensory integration, there are several sensory systems of concern. One of the earliest to mature is the vestibular system. This system of balance and posture provides information about movement and gravitational pull. Children with fragile X frequently present with behaviors and responses to their environment that indicate abnormal processing of vestibular information. A person's system may be underresponsive, overreactive, or fluctuate between these two extremes depending on the situation (Anderson, 1992).

Another important and early maturing sensory system is the kinesthetic/proprioceptive system. It provides information on touch and body position. Nerve endings for this system are found in muscles, tendons, joints, and skin. With the exception of muscles, these tissues are all connective tissue, which may be the reason this system is so often disordered in a child with fra(X). When this system is functioning well, incoming information is accurately interpreted and guides the rest of the central nervous system in providing awareness of location of the body and its parts in space. Information about how the body is positioned with respect to other people or objects around it is also provided.

The importance of the vestibular and kinesthetic/proprioceptive systems in concert is that they provide appropriate balance (against gravity and during movement). If a person does not have good balance reactions, good quality of movement will not be present either. The person feels unsafe and insecure. The two systems in concert also provide a sense of being organized and knowing one's place within the environment even when that environment changes. These are feelings crucial to a sense of well-being and security. The person with fra(X) whose vestibular and kinesthetic/proprioceptive systems are not functioning normally is apt not to feel secure, organized, or in control of him- or herself. In seeking to achieve those feelings, Anderson (1992) suggests that some of the aberrant or so-called self-stimulatory behaviors noted in boys with fra(X) may be their attempts to create a sense of well-being for themselves. The behaviors any one child latches onto for himself can vary, but they will be rhythmical and repetitive. One bit of evidence that these behaviors may soothe is their increased occurrence when the child is upset or anxious. Further discussion of anxiety associated with fra(X) is provided in the section on emotional aspects related to the syndrome.

Tactile information must be adequately and efficiently processed and integrated into the child's image of how he or she fits into the social and physical surroundings. An impaired tactile system can be hyper-reactive, hyporeactive, or alternate between the two extremes. Males and females with fra(X) frequently are hyper-reactive to several kinds of input, including tactile. This condition, called tactile defensiveness, may be evident during infancy. Fragile X babies frequently are irritable and may intensely protest about daily care which involves much handling and exposure of body parts to changing sensations. Infants and children with tactile defensivity may not be cuddly. A defensive reaction to touch will be elicited by a light touch from other people or objects, such as a breeze or blades of grass. It may also be a response to certain textures and temperatures. Hands, feet, and the inside of the mouth are some of the most sensitive locations for anyone, but especially for people with fra(X). Oral hypersensitivity will be treated more fully under the section on oral sensory and motor aspects.

A person with tactile defensiveness is commonly also hypersensitive to other incoming stimuli through the modalities of vision, hearing, taste, and smell. Estimates range as high as 90% of individuals with the disorder who have poor eye contact. In fact, the poor eye contact and the purposeful gaze aversion so often mentioned with fra(X) may be hypersensitive responses to other people. In social interactions, people do considerable moving and changing with their bodies, especially their faces, in ways that are filled with meaning for most people. The amount and rate of changing information may be overwhelming to the processing capabilities of the person with fra(X). Clinically, the child may be observed trying to block out stimulation that feels overwhelming and produces anxiety or a sense of being out of control. The child may cover his or her ears, eyes, nose, or mouth, or avert his or her eyes until a feeling of control is regained or the offending stimulus goes away. Other possible reactions include acting out, withdrawing from the situation, or using repetitive body movements.

Imagine being distracted or set on edge by sights, sounds, smells, or touch that are part of one's daily environment, things that are disregarded by most people. A child who cannot ignore them is constantly having his attention, ability to learn from events, and communication interrupted. In other words, the fra(X) child who is hypersensitive may miss important input while feeling assaulted by what everyone else considers inconsequential phenomena. Another result of being hypersensitive to touch is that the child may not like the feel of objects in his or her hand. Fine motor and visual motor skills cannot develop normally if the child cannot tolerate holding handles, tools, lids, or other things long enough to learn how to work with them.

An area of learning and development often affected by the sensory integration dysfunction of fra(X) is the ability to visually orient oneself in the environment, recognize the spatial relationship of objects, and integrate pieces of visual information to form the gestalt. This is an area of deficit often seen in females with fra(X) as well as in males. It may be one of the few characteristics related to the genetic disorder that a female demonstrates. Its occurrence seems unrelated to the rest of her cognitive picture. Left-right disorientation is one expression of the deficit that the girls often show.

With poor visual-spatial ability, a child does not have a good sense of where and how he or she fits into the surroundings. There is no basis for moving around in space or for manipulating nearby objects. Familiar surroundings will seem like new ones when something is changed (e.g., if the child usually goes to the media center with a group but now enters alone). Visual motor tasks are affected so that activities such as drawing, writing, or putting puzzles together are made more difficult.

The many ways a child with fra(X) is unable to adequately and accurately integrate incoming sensory information from the several modalities can be overwhelming. Indeed, this is how children with fra(X) often present, as being easily overstimulated which, depending on the child, may result in tantrums, repetitive movements, or withdrawing. Some children reach the point of self-injurious behavior. Those who have developed language may use it perseveratively at these times.

Attention and Activity Level

A child with the diagnosis of fra(X) is also more likely than usual to receive a diagnosis of attention deficit disorder, especially with hyperactivity. The majority of boys with fra(X), as many as 90%, have also been diagnosed ADD (Hagerman, Kemper, & Hudson, 1985), as have many of the girls with the syndrome (Hagerman, 1992). Like others with that diagnosis, these children are impulsive, easily overstimulated, distractible, have trouble making transitions between activities, and may be exceptionally overactive. For example, one 4-year-old watches his favorite TV shows with rapt attention while he runs and jumps around the room riding a hobby horse. Techniques for calming and quieting will be discussed in the section on treatment. Medication for treating ADD is successful with many children also diagnosed as having the fra(X) syndrome.

Cognitive and Learning Characteristics

Knowing a boy has fragile X provides little information about his level of cognitive functioning. He may function within the normal range, often with learning disabilities, or he may show impairment to the severe range of mental retardation. From what we know thus far, it appears that most males with fra(X) have a level of cognitive functioning in the range of mild to moderate retardation. Researchers are finding that fra(X) males perform more poorly on tasks that require sequential processing and on tasks of arithmetic knowledge than boys without fra(X). The research also supports earlier reports that boys with fra(X) often function better in daily life and do better academically than their intelligence scores would predict (McClennen, 1992). There is also suggestion in the literature that some boys show a decline in scores on standardized measures of intelligence as they get older. The reason for this decline, as well as any delineation of a subgroup of children in which this can be expected, is unclear. Batshaw, Perret, and Shapiro (1992) speculated that, in those cases, the child's nonverbal skills were overestimated at earlier ages.

Professionals should be aware of additional information that exists on learning and learning style in planning for a child with fra(X). Just as with other forms of mental retardation, a retarded child with fra(X) will require labeling, highlighting, practicing, and focus on learning some skills that age peers learn on their own without instruction. In general, the child will learn more slowly and do better with more concrete than abstract concepts such that critical thinking, flexibility in thinking, and problem-solving are difficult. The ability to generalize information in a new way or to a new situation is also likely to be impaired. Storing and retrieving information, as well as focusing or shifting attention, are predicted areas of difficulty for the child with fra(X) as for other children with mental retardation.

The ability to learn information presented sequentially is another area of particular weakness for the child with fra(X), just as it is for children with Down syndrome. This difficulty has been found to occur whether the task involves a situation from standardized testing, something the child encounters in daily life, or an academic task. Visual and auditory sequencing are difficulties fairly typical of females with fra(X) as well.

Boys with fra(X) and retardation differ in some ways from children with retardation due to other causes. Research has indicated that many people, male and female, with fra(X) learn more quickly and easily through the visual modality than through the auditory modality. Their best visual skills are seeing the whole, or gestalt, and having memory for visual information. Researchers have suggested that these factors may be important in accounting for why the child with fra(X) learns reading and spelling more easily than would be predicted by his or her standardized test scores.

As noted earlier, girls with fra(X) often perform within the normal range on measures of intelligence. Of all girls receiving a diagnosis of fra(X), about 25% will have IQ scores below 70, and 25% will be in the borderline normal range of intelligence (Scharfenaker, 1990). Regardless of where their scores fall, girls with fra(X) tend to show most weakness in the concepts underlying math and in abstract reasoning. Although in general their visual skills dominate their auditory skills, they still may be weak in visual-spatial processing of information. On standardized measures of intelligence, they may be expected to have the most difficulty with the subtests of block design, arithmetic, and digit span.

Speech, Oral Sensory and Motor, and Language Characteristics

The range of possible speech and language deficits associated with fragile X is quite wide. The child may have only slight difficulty with abstract reasoning. This very mild level of impairment occurs more often in girls with fra(X) than in boys. At the other end of the range, a child may have significant deficits in language, speech, and voice. Most children diagnosed with fra(X) have some, but not all, of the identified deficits. Girls more closely match boys in disorders of speech and language abilities than they do in other areas of development.

As noted earlier, children with fra(X) often have significant problems processing sensory information. In particular, many of them are hypersensitive to facial and oral stimulation from food, the articulators, implements for hygiene, and touch. The same child can be hyposensitive as well, and be unaware of small bits of food in or around his mouth, unaware that he is drooling, and unaware of where his tongue is touching inside his mouth. At a later age, the child may continue to show pooling of saliva especially during extended speech and during fine motor tasks using his hands.

Professionals have found that boys with fragile X usually show oral sensory and motor deficits for both feeding and speech production. These are children who can have mild to severe problems with feeding beginning in infancy. As infants, some of these children do not have an efficient suck due to their poor sensory feedback and hypotonia. Therefore, they may be very slow feeders (Lowe, 1992). Depending on when intervention begins, and on the aspects of foods to which they react negatively, this group of children can have very limited diets. Mealtime can be a source of stress for the entire family. Tactile defensiveness can also lead to unusual ways of eating, for example, for a child who cannot tolerate oral or manual contact with utensils. A child like this may, for example, accept a quick bite from a spoon while turning away. The child may refuse to hold a utensil at the expected age and level of ability. Clearly, these issues build on each other. As a result, the child is less independent and misses the feeling of mastery of a new tool. Changes in feeding routine, already a source of anxiety, add still more stress and can leave the child feeling irritable. This makes meals an unpleasant time for the whole family.

Just as with any child with tactile hypersensitivities, a young child with a diagnosis of fra(X) may refuse to even try a food that looks different from the familiar. Altering even a familiar and well-liked food (e.g., by trying to hide mashed green beans in mashed potatoes) can lead to refusal to get near the food and to frustration about not being able to eat.

Tactile hypersensitivity also often affects hygiene. Depending on the child, bathing or washing and shampooing around face and head may not be easily tolerated. Teeth-brushing or an approaching tissue can lead to a huge upset. Parents may end up doing the minimum amount of bathing and cleaning possible to avoid conflicts ensuing. For these children, teeth-brushing, in particular, often is eliminated from the daily routine because it is such a battle.

Along with oral tactile defensiveness, the child with fra(X) is likely to be hypotonic and have lax joints. Both will have an impact on the development and quality of feeding abilities and on speech production. Therapists familiar with oral sensory and motor development will notice a delayed ability to keep the jaw stable during the motor tasks of eating and speech. The child will have a difficult time getting lingual movements disassociated from the jaw and using those movements in a rapid and efficient way for speech. Generally children with fra(X) are delayed in the age at which speech begins. After it does start, there will often be remaining delays in articulation. Because of all these problems, the child may continue to show a breakdown in articulatory capability for connected speech. Multiword utterances require long sequences of rapid movements, and the speaker must still make the contact points adequately.

The hypotonia, loose joints, and poor processing of the proprioceptive information coming from oral sensors may be why children with fra(X) sometimes use prolonged and frequent mouthing and biting on their own fingers and hands, and on nonfood objects. Schopmeyer (1992) noted that this may be related to the serious self-biting sometimes seen in fra(X) boys with more severe cognitive impairment and autism. Just as with young, typically developing children, there may also be a need for the comfort aspect derived from sucking and mouthing things. The added biting down on objects seen in children with fra(X) may stem from their need to have external help to stabilize the jaw.

Breakdown in intelligibility of speech in connected passages is frequently seen in children with fragile X. The underlying motor and sensory picture for children with fra(X) has been described. Along with difficulty making articulatory contacts quickly and concisely enough, the child with fra(X) often uses an excessively rapid rate of speech. Rate also increases with anxiety, and high anxiety is another prominent feature of fra(X). Several researchers have noted a cluttering quality to speech for both boys and girls. Children have frequent syllable repetitions, false starts, rapid and irregular rate, and breakdowns in syntax. Cluttering is another feature associated with fra(X) that worsens with increased anxiety. Some professionals have found dyspraxia in association with fra(X). It has been noted that there is often a delay in vowel acquisition for words. Multisyllabic words are especially difficult for the child with fra(X) (Schopmeyer, 1992).

Finally, the amount of retardation has been found to correlate with the articulation ability of the child.

Voice quality in boys with fra(X) has been characterized as hoarse, breathy, and low in pitch. Loudness may or may not be affected in any consistent way. Girls who have an abnormal voice quality associated with fra(X) seem to have a higher than normal pitch (Reiss & Freund, 1990). There are also findings that intonation, stress, and juncture are rhythmic features disordered by fra(X) (Schopmeyer, 1992).

All of these characteristics, often in addition to inadequate articulation, poor eye contact, body orientation, and rapid rate, contribute to poor intelligibility in connected speech. The reasons for some of these things are not known. It is possible that the vocal qualities result from hypotonia. Lowe (1992) speculated that the dyspraxia evident in some of the children makes it difficult for them to coordinate and order the sequence of movements for respiration, voicing, and articulation together with language. Anxiety could be a factor as well.

Several aspects of fra(X) syndrome can interfere with processing receptive language. The child with poor attention can be distracted before incoming information is securely processed and stored. As with other children with disordered attention, when something is of great interest to them, they show better comprehension and memory for it. In addition, the heightened level of anxiety associated with fra(X) makes adequate concentration less likely. The hypersensitivity to gaze experienced by many children with fra(X) deprives them of visual information a listener ordinarily gets from watching a speaker's mouth, face, and body during communication. Remember that many individuals with fra(X) have some level of lowered cognitive ability which affects language comprehension as well. And, finally, the processing of language may in and of itself be disordered for some boys and girls with fra(X).

The expressive language of children with fra(X) often has several features which professionals have noted to be characteristic of the syndrome. For example, one characteristic frequently observed is the use of the gestalt, or language "chunk" approach to learning language. These children learn new phrases as part of situations more often than they add words to classes such as verbs or prepositions. The chunks learned are used, for the most part, in appropriate contexts. The children eventually apply the grammar rules contained in what they have learned to additional words and contexts, increasing their expressive repertoire. How far the child's language develops in syntactic complexity and content will be very much dependent on cognitive level.

Echolalia is another feature often listed as characteristic of the language of children with fragile X (Schopmeyer, 1992). This is more frequently found in the expressive language of those with the additional diagnosis of autism, but it also is seen in individuals with no autism and little retardation as well. Delayed echolalia makes sense in light of initial language learning in the gestalt style. Pronominal reversals are not usually reported as part of echolalia associated with fra(X), and the words or phrases echoed are often interjections (e.g., "alright!" or "I used my brain!" derived from "You used your brain!" as praise for the child working at learning tasks).

Perseveration in verbal expression is also considered characteristic of the language of boys and some girls having fra(X). The perseverative language is generally used in the appropriate context and also seems at times to be used to elicit reactions from others. For a child with disorganized, cluttered expression, using a word or phrase over and over may be an easy way of sharing thoughts, feelings, and interests and getting verbal responses from others. Word retrieval is another aspect of language that is impaired by fra(X) syndrome. The use of echolalia and the perseveration on a topic or language unit may be a result of anxiety and inadequate word retrieval having their impact on the child's communication attempts.

Some professionals have commented on the volume of expressive language coming from individuals with fra(X) (Schopmeyer, 1992). This is not true for all individuals, nor in every situation, considering the anxiety, dyspraxia, hypersensitivities, and other issues. Maintaining a topic is a conversational skill that many individuals with fra(X) find difficult. Volubility and inadequate topic maintenance are sometimes observed in people diagnosed with ADD. They seem unable to gate anything coming into their minds from putting it into words. In addition, poor word retrieval or poor expressive organization make getting to the point difficult. In people with fra(X), talking is directed both toward themselves and others. Perhaps because of the ADD component, they too easily leave one topic for tangential information. But coupled with the large amount of talking coming from a person also diagnosed with fra(X) the lack of topic maintenance is a more prominent feature.

Autism is a severe communication disorder. Pervasive Developmental Disorder (PDD) is a less severe form on the same continuum of communication disorder (see Chapter 7, Autism and PDD). These disorders occur in about 15% of the children identified as having fragile X syndrome. Most of the 15% are males. Along with fra(X) and autism, these are usually the children with the greatest degree of mental retardation and disordered integration of sensory information, including that coming through the auditory channel.

Emotional Characteristics

The hallmark of the emotional profile observed by many professionals studying fragile X is the high level of social anxiety the people with fra(X) seem to feel. Gaze avoidance and body orientation away from others is typical of individuals with fra(X), even when encountering familiar people in familiar situations. However, gaze avoidance does not ordinarily happen with a child's parents or significant others (Lowe, 1992). Social situations have been observed to provoke anxiety for boys with fra(X), even when the situation is familiar and the child is part of a group. Girls with fra(X) are typically characterized as timid. The source of their high level of anxiety is unclear, but it has an impact on many of the behaviors and abilities we have been discussing. The anxiety is thought to be at least partly responsible for the stereotypies and self-biting observed in some children with fra(X) as well as the cluttering and perseveration. Perhaps the anxiety is related to the children's hypersensitivities, because it also is characteristic of other children with sensory integration dysfunction including hypersensitivities.

Some girls with fra(X) are socially anxious to the point of being diagnosed as having Avoidant Disorder in childhood or adolescence, that is to say, the girls avoid unfamiliar people to a degree that handicaps their ability to form peer relationships. Girls with fra(X) were also more likely than peers to experience social and emotional disturbance as adolescents (Freund, 1991).

Despite the anxiety social situations appear to evoke in these children, many still have a great interest in their peers. For example, one 4-year-old loved his preschool classmates and looked forward to seeing them each day. Yet his way of approaching other children was to run around them, not stopping, not getting close, and not saying anything. Goals for this child's IEP would need to include approaching, but not touching others, using specific phrases to initiate interactions, using appropriate eye contact, and so on.

Strengths Typical of the Child with Fragile X

Although the child may have the communicative deficits we have discussed, a child with fra(X) is often thought of by others as engaging and sociable. Parents, especially, often describe the child with words such as "sweet" and "loving." Children with fra(X) want to please the adults who are important in their lives. Although they may not understand how to approach and interact with peers, they show a great interest in peer interactions. To this end, they may seek ways to contact other children. Their interest in others, along with their good imitative abilities, make them good candidates for inclusion programs. With appropriate models they can learn to develop better social skills. Individuals with fra(X) have often been found to have a great interest in music. This indicates a direction parents might pursue for social development, language and sensory integration development, and as a good leisure activity for their children. A good sense of humor is observed by many professionals and parents alike. Although abstract humor would likely not be of interest, children with fra(X) enjoy more slapstick sort of comedy such as clowns. Basically, they are cheerful people and have a ready laugh. All of this makes them very pleasant people to be around.

Assessment

Because the fragile X disorder affects so many areas of learning and development, as well as having physical and emotional consequences, it is vital that a child be diagnosed as early as possible. Knowing the possible impairments associated with fra(X) and making an assessment or monitoring for them enables the child and family to get the help they need. Early intervention can lessen some aspects of the disorder with which the child and family will struggle. Perhaps it can also prevent misunderstandings about the child's behavior (e.g., in the case of the child with tactile hypersensitivities). The other major reason for the earliest possible diagnosis is to indicate the need for genetic testing of other family members. Prospective parents need to be able to make informed decisions about whether or not to have children given their particular chances of passing the syndrome on to their children. It can be a great relief for parents, and individuals with fra(X) themselves, to have a reason for learning disabilities, attentional deficits, hypersensitivities, and so on.

The best avenue of assessment for individuals with the diagnosis is through a team of professionals with expertise in social-emotional growth, cognition (including an understanding of executive function), attention and behavior, speech, language, oral sensory and motor development, gross and fine motor growth, and sensory integration. Of course, medical examination to look for any of the problems listed earlier should be done or may have been the way the child was suspected of having the fra(X) condition in the first place. Audiology, neurology, and ophthalmology are other disciplines in which assessments are needed as early as possible to look for any existing problems.

The diagnosis of fragile X should be made by genetics assessment only. However, professionals in Child Find, Head Start, early intervention programs, and clinics for speech and language can be the first to notice characteristics pointing to fra(X). All the professionals involved in assessing a child need a knowledge of fra(X) features. They must know the problems or issues that need to be addressed, monitored, or assessed further as the individual gets older. All of the professionals involved also need an awareness of the continuum of severity that fra(X) can produce for any given area of growth, learning, or development. The disorder includes a wide range of severity. Therefore, each professional needs to keep an open mind so as not to limit a child's possible progress. It also is important to keep in mind the strengths often found in persons with fra(X) and look at how they might be useful for each person. Individual strengths can help the learning process along, provide a basis for communication, and build a sense of competence and self-esteem.

Professionals who work with children with fra(X) syndrome have observed that, as a general rule, the children do not perform on standardized assessment tasks commensurate with how well they perform in daily situations (McClennen, 1992). McClennen cites the example that children with fra(X) seem to show better auditory and visual memory in real situations than their scores on standardized measures would indicate. It has been suggested that the children's high anxiety level as a group might be why this is so. Context also seems a likely reason. If these children learn primarily in a gestalt manner, taking something out of context, or asking for a new, unpracticed behavior or demonstration of knowledge, would not be a good measure of how easily they typically learn.

Along with, or as part of the reason for, increased anxiety, many individuals with fra(X) have attention deficits and hyperactivity. Children with these disorders often have difficulty with the high level of structure, heavy linguistic demands, and repetitive nature of standardized tasks. In addition, word-retrieval difficulties are common among those with fra(X) so that "on demand" recall out of context often does not work well with these children (Schopmeyer, 1992).

With all of the indications that standardized tests may not present a child's best ability in the area under assessment, clinicians may want to alter the test situation or task, after using the standard procedure, to get more information on the child's level of knowledge. Another possibility is to use curriculum-based assessment and classroom and home observations. Under what circumstances can the child do the task or use the information?

In trying to determine the child's best level of function, most information may come from observation in the child's daily routine and when the child initiates an activity on his or her own. Even under the most comfortable routine circumstances, the child with fra(X) may not be able to answer direct questions or follow direct requests to do things he or she spontaneously does.

Treatment

Although people with fragile X have some aspects of impairment in common, as individuals each has his or her own unique strengths and areas of weakness for learning and development. Some factors that will affect the long-term outcome of each person's development in general and his or her communication capability specifically are the degree of expression of the fra(X) characteristics, the degree of cognitive impairment, the presence of behavioral issues, and disordered sensory integration.

Batshaw, Perret, and Shapiro (1992) reported that the literature on the controversial treatment of administering doses of folic acid to those with fra(X) has not shown efficacy for improving behavior or the ability to learn. Others, such as Hagerman (1992), feel it does improve attention and language development in some children.

Medication is often used successfully to treat the ADD component of fra(X) as well as the aggressive behavior sometimes seen as the children grow into adolescence and adulthood. As for other children with attention deficits and hyperactivity, stimulant medications do not work for all. They are found useful for about two thirds to three quarters of children identified as having fra(X) syndrome. However, children with fra(X) may be more sensitive to the medications and can show mood and behavior disruptions at lower doses than might otherwise be expected. Tricyclic antidepressant drugs and other categories of drugs are also being used to treat attention deficits. Children with fra(X) seem more sensitive to these medications as well (Hagerman,1992).

The best and most complete intervention is to identify, assess, and begin treatment in an appropriate developmental program as early as possible.

Infancy

There are several areas of development that can be recognized as already impaired in infancy by the fra(X) genetic condition. Some of these can pose serious threats to the child's well-being because they affect how he or she interacts with caregivers and the environment at this early age.

Even in early infancy a baby with fra(X) may have problems achieving and maintaining a calm alert state because of poorly developed systems of touch, kinesthesis and proprioception, and balance. The parents will find such a child to be easily overstimulated, frequently irritable, perhaps not happy to be held and snuggled, nor bathed and changed. Additionally, oral hypersensitivity may make feeding difficult and unpleasant for everyone involved. If low muscle tone exists, the child's capability for sucking and eventual food management may be inadequate.

Early intervention involves teaching the caregivers about the child's difficulties so that they realize that the problem is not that they are not good enough parents nor that their child does not like them. Nor is the child being demanding for no good reason. Show them how to keep stimulation to a minimum and let them know that a consistent routine will help the child regulate attentional states. Explain how they can read their infant's cues as to when he or she is available or has had enough. Make suggestions for environmental factors (e.g., the use of soothing music, soft lighting, water temperature for bathing, etc.) to avoid overwhelming the infant's fragile nervous system. Teach calming techniques of swaddling the baby in a blanket with his hands at midline, using a pacifier and rocking vertically for appropriate vestibular stimulation. Touch should be firm and, especially around the baby's mouth, hands, and feet, and it should be slow and gradual to reduce hypersensitivity. Teach the parents why feeding is so difficult and have them allow extra time if necessary. The parents need information on handling techniques individualized for their child's hypotonia and lax joints along with any exercises or types of stimulation they should provide. When solid foods are to be introduced along with feeding utensils, parents need to be prepared to respond to the child rejecting these changes in routine. They need to know how to make the changes as gradual and as easy as possible, but also realize that the child *must* make those transitions. The clinician can communicate to the parents that delaying the changes will cause the child to reject them even more strenuously at a later age. They need help to avoid the development of negative behaviors that will grow worse with time, and be willing to stay with the process until the child can adjust.

Toddlers and Preschoolers

Children with fra(X) are generally gestalt language learners. Therefore, they are less likely to encounter difficulty with the memorized aspects of English (e.g., irregular past tenses, changing from object to subject pronouns, etc.). Difficulty is more likely to occur in extracting the rules underlying grammar and morphology, such as adding -s to verbs for the third person singular present tense.

Hypotonicity and lax joints along with hyposensitivity (which can co-occur with hypersensitivity) mean that a young child with fra(X) can be a profuse drooler. If this continues to be an issue at 3 to 4 years of age and beyond, continue to work on strengthening muscles and giving the joints extra deep stimulation. Simultaneously, work to improve the child's awareness of wetness and provide a socially appropriate method for managing saliva. Have the child wear a sweatband on his or her wrist for wiping. These are available in children's sizes. In the preschool years, it is still socially appropriate to have the child use the cuff of a sleeve or the shirt neckband. These children also may stuff their mouths too full of food as a result of hyposensitivity and hypotonia. A too full mouth leaves the child unable to manage the food adequately and allows no room to learn to use the tongue for manipulating and keeping track of the food. A mirror works well for these children during a snack (not at family mealtime or when the child is very hungry). With a mirror the child can see what you mean when told "your mouth is/is not ready" or "your tongue needs to clean up its room." Teach the child to eat "regular" not "monster" sized bites.

In this age range, questions may arise as to whether attention deficits and hyperactivity are present. Delays in reaching developmental milestones will have begun to appear by this point. Issues of sensory integration dysfunction, if present, will have been underway for some time so that the child may have developed some idiosyncratic ways of organizing, providing, or shutting out stimulation to meet the needs of his or her nervous system. As with the younger child, it is important to provide as much external structure as necessary so that, through practice, the child can begin to develop an internal sense of structure. An individual plan for treatment should include play groups or more structured programs including typically developing children as models for communication and social behavior. The clinician should take advantage of the good imitation skills and high social interest the child with fra(X) will probably have. Use an auditory trainer or similar device providing low-level amplification along with earphones for improving the signal-to-noise ratio during therapy sessions, when the child is read to, and so on. This technique is especially helpful for children with attention deficits and disordered auditory processing. It also works well for any child who needs to focus on sounds or aspects of grammar, vocabulary, or concepts.

Children with fra(X) are often late in beginning to use their first words. In many cases, there is a significant discrepancy between their receptive and expressive language skills early on. For this reason, children with fra(X) can be good candidates for using augmentative communication systems. Both manual sign and language boards, or a combination of the two, will work for toddlers and preschoolers before they begin using words, while their vocabularies are building up, and to augment preschoolers' ability to combine words. Manual sign particularly can continue to be of use receptively long after a child has dropped its use in favor of spoken words. Signs serve well to augment inadequate language processing as well as for cues regarding grammatical morphemes the child is learning to use.

Once the child with fra(X) acquires some expressive language, he or she may use it in great volume. McClennen (1992) suggests putting the expressive language to work in augmenting inadequate receptive language processing and attention deficits. The child with fra(X) can rehearse directions given while carrying them out. The child can also talk him- or herself through a series of activities where memory typically interferes (e.g., putting work away and getting ready for lunch). McClennen further suggests translating visual information into words. One example of this would be having the child with fra(X) describe the pictures in a book that the teacher is reading to the group.

In the classroom, use of visual and manipulative representations of activities is a good way to establish the routine and make transitions within it. The child with fra(X) needs one-to-one and small group instruction as much as possible for learning new information so that maximum attention is maintained. As with other children with attention deficits, the child with fra(X) will need well-defined learning or activity stations with clear boundaries. Whenever possible, using enclosures to block other visual and auditory activities can help maintain attention to task. It is also helpful to establish a quiet place where a child can go to pull him- or herself together. Depending on the need, it may contain a place for sprawling or getting cozy. It may provide rhythmic movement (rocking, swinging, or bouncing) or there may be earphones and music or story tapes.

Providing models to imitate is important for children with fra(X) across several realms of activities, including gross motor (learning to ride a bike by watching other children) and fine motor (learning to hook train cars together by perhaps watching others do it and hand-over-hand instruction if necessary). The child will learn appropriate words and phrases by direct instruction along with models using the language needed for an activity. Kaye (1992) says also that children with fra(X) learn best by seeing the result of a completed activity at the beginning. This way they have a concrete image to follow because trying to imagine where a step in a project is leading is not easy for them. The child also needs to complete an activity before answering questions about it.

The clinician for a child with fragile X needs to be mindful of seating for play, listening, group participation, and eating. A child with hypotonia, lax joints, and inadequate sensory integration will need external support for stability. Stability provides the basis from which speech, eating, and other fine motor activities can occur, and helps the child feel secure in space. External support can also reduce assaults on the child's hypersensitivities (Kaye, 1992).

Many children with communication disorders need to develop better social eye contact. If, as many experts feel, the inadequate eye contact observed in children with fra(X) stems from anxiety and hypersensitivity, improving it will require a gentle approach. Eye contact should be treated like any other skill the child has not yet developed. Ask for it and provide praise when it occurs. Gradually work up to longer intervals. The clinician should alert the child before looking directly at him or her.

School Age and Beyond

Kaye (1992) suggests teaching a child with fra(X) to give him- or herself firm pressure on the skin and deep pressure into joints. Children with this disorder need deeper pressure than normal to feel in control and secure in relation to the physical and social environment. This author suggests having the child push down on his or her own head and into joints by doing chair push-ups, pushing on a table or against a wall, and rocking on all fours. At younger ages, the adult will initiate or direct the child to do these things, but at older ages a child can learn to monitor his own feelings and behavior and learn cues that signal when to do these things. The child can initiate the deep pressure activities as stress rises or when he or she feels out of control. These exercises could also be used *after* a time of stress. For example, a 5-year-old may have as a goal on his IEP that he will begin monitoring his feelings and behavior and recognize when he is getting out of control or anxious. He could be taught to ask for time in a bean bag or rocking chair whenever he recognizes the negative feelings arising.

Children with fra(X) who have attention deficits, hyperactivity, and problems integrating sensory information may need a lot of leeway in how they are best able to listen and attend. These children will need more frequent breaks. They may not look as if they *could* be attending because they may not be giving eye contact to the speaker, their bodies may be oriented away from the speaker, or they may be up and moving around (McClennen, 1992). They may *need* to move around (maybe in a chair or piece of equipment). For example, a child may need to do structured activities from a rocking chair. That way the child can move, yet stay in control and attentive. Carrels or dividers can provide a sense of enclosure and security. Children with fra(X) may attend best while listening through headphones with an auditory trainer. Because of hypersensitivity to interpersonal eye contact, children with fra(X) may need to be seated where they do not face other students or the teacher (Kaye,1992).

For many children with fra(X), learning to read is probably best done primarily through a sight word approach rather than by learning phonics rules and applying them to reading. Experience suggests that, although these children may learn the sound-symbol relationships, their poor auditory sequencing may prevent them from learning to sound out words for reading and spelling (McClennen,1992).

Computers can be a good tool for teaching children with fra(X), just as they are for the typically developing child. Computers are especially useful for children with fra(X) for several reasons. First, the graphics and the fun of pushing buttons or moving pieces of equipment and seeing changes on the screen make children feel successful and empowered. Second, computers have been found particularly useful for children with attention deficits. They function as tools that can provide the excitement and changes in presentation that seem to work best for children with attention deficits. Additionally, these children eventually may need to do written work on the computer to circumvent fine motor deficits.

Case Management Issues

There are several issues to keep in mind when seeing a child with fra(X) syndrome. One issue that may arise is the discrepancy between the child's performance at home and in school. With the social anxiety and performance pressure many children with fra(X) present, as well as being creatures of routine and performing best in the situation in which learning occurred, these are children for whom there often is a discrepancy between performance at home or with family versus in early intervention and school programs. Parents can easily feel frustrated when their child cannot perform in school. Care needs to be taken to ensure that they do not feel staff think they are exaggerating about their child's abilities. The staff members, for their part, have to know that the child may not be showing all he or she knows. An appropriate goal for intervention then becomes helping the child generalize performance at home to the school setting.

Another issue involves the ethical responsibility the professional working with the child and family holds to provide current and accurate information regarding the child's disorder. This includes what is known of the genetic inheritance of fra(X) syndrome and of the child's language and speech disorders. The parents should receive information about the heritable nature of fra(X), and it is incumbent on involved professionals to try to see that the information is adequately understood. The parents as well as other family members need to have the information necessary to make informed choices regarding having additional children as well as the need for relatives not of the nuclear family to get genetic testing.

Professionals working with older children who seem to fit the characteristics of fra(X) but who have not been genetically tested need to be ready to refer parents back to the pediatrician with the question of whether genetic testing needs to be done. The existence of fra(X) is too recently known and too poorly recognized in individuals for clinicians to assume that an older child or adolescent must surely have been tested already.

A great many children with fra(X) syndrome have inadequate processing of auditory information, often as part of a more global sensory integration dysfunction. Therefore, these children will be considered by some professionals to be appropriate candidates for auditory integration training (AIT) (also referred to as Auditory Enhancement Training [AET] or Audio-Psycho-Phonology). AIT is believed by its practitioners to improve processing of environmental sounds and speech, thereby affecting a wide range of abilities and behaviors, including receptive and expressive language, attention, hyperacusis, hypoacusis, behavioral aggression, and poor self-image, among others. At this point, the American Speech-Language-Hearing Association has recommended that parents considering the use of AIT be told that it is experimental and that there is not conclusive, scientific data to support its use at this time. The Food and Drug Administration, in September 1993, banned the further import of one device used to administer AIT pending further investigation of its use and efficacy (ASHA Ad Hoc Committee on Auditory Integration and Facilitated Communication, 1994).

Summary

Fragile X syndrome is a disorder causing a wide range of effects from mild to severe across multiple possible areas of physiology, anatomy, learning, development, and behavior. There is a need to improve the accuracy and timeliness of diagnosis so that the appropriate interventions for individual children can begin as early as possible. Fra(X) presents numerous obstacles for a child and his or her family, but with support, they can be surmounted and the child can make gains toward independence, health, and a happy life.

CHAPTER 5

Neglect and Abuse

Definition and Incidence

An estimated 1 in every 10 children has been abused or neglected. Although these children have not been identified as a specific population eligible for special education services under Public Law 99-457, many will meet the criteria for service as at-risk children for inclusion in classes for the emotionally disturbed, language impaired, learning disabled, and mentally handicapped.

Defining the different types of child maltreatment is a difficult task. There is considerable controversy over this issue because the nature of maltreatment of children does not lend itself to indisputable definitions that will apply to each and every new situation that develops. In addition, various definitions may be adopted by organizations, government, communities, and individuals to serve a certain purpose. For example, social workers who investigate accusations of maltreatment may not rely solely on a legally based definition which focuses on evidential criteria to prove the act of abuse. They will evaluate other factors including family resources and the child's need for protection to determine whether or not abuse has occurred.

The National Committee on Child Abuse defines maltreatment of children as falling into one of four categories: physical abuse, sexual abuse, emotional maltreatment, and neglect. Physical abuse includes the shaking, beating, burning, and poisoning of the child that results in bodily injury and/or lasting neurological damage. Although legal definitions of child abuse rely heavily on the overt consequences of the abuse (e.g., bruises, welts, etc.), they serve an important purpose in identifying the minimum community standards for child care (Wolfe, 1987).

Sexual abuse, which is on the rise, includes the involvement of the child in any sexual act or situation including incest, exploitation, intercourse, molestation, nonphysical indecent exposure, and verbal attacks that are of a sexual nature (Trace, 1992; Wolfe, 1987).

Emotional maltreatment refers to behavior by the caretaker that causes low self-esteem of the child, undue fear or anxiety, or other damage to the child's emotional well-being. This type of maltreatment can include excessive teasing or yelling at the child, in addition to failure to provide essential attention and affection for the child (Trace, 1992; Wolfe, 1987).

The final category is neglect, which is sometimes difficult to identify. Neglect involves failure on the part of the caretaker to provide proper nutrition, clothing, shelter, personal hygiene, or medical care. This area also involves inadequate supervision of the child for extended lengths of time. Frequently the child is left at home alone for long periods of time at an early age or is left with a child who is too young for supervisory responsibilities. Among all types of maltreated children, those who are neglected are most prone to developing communication characteristics of neglected and abused children disorders.

Risk Factors

Many studies have been conducted to evaluate the effects of environmental influences on cognitive development. These studies have reported that there is a relationship between family social status and the child's intellectual performance (Culp et al., 1991; Hoff-Ginsberg, 1989) Low socioeconomic status (SES) has been found to have a negative effect on mother-child interactions. Studies evaluating social status have documented that children from disadvantaged homes generally experience decreased opportunities for verbal interaction and often do not experience the type of verbal input necessary for cognitive and linguistic competence (Cicchetti, 1990; Cohen & Beckwith, 1974).

Mothers from low SES generally are less stimulating and less responsive to the child, less sophisticated in language use, more restrictive and controlling in behavior, and use less descriptive language (Barnes, Gutfreund, Satterly, & Wells, 1983; Culp, Watkins, Lawrence, Letts, Kelly, & Rice, 1991; Hoff-Ginsberg, 1989; Mash, Johnston, & Kovitz, 1983).

Much research to date supports the fact that the characteristics of the language environment and the nature of the parent-infant interaction have definite effects on the child's development of cognitive and linguistic skills. Children who are engaged in stimulating interactions as infants develop strong cognitive abilities, language, and social skills. Children who are under the influence of parental input that is highly controlling and directive in nature show decreased cognitive and linguistic development (Snow, Midkiff-Borundo, Small, & Proctor, 1984).

The investigation of parent-child attachment in maltreated infants has made significant contributions in the understanding of relationship formation as well as the risk factors contributing to child maltreatment. Bell and Ainsworth (1972) reported that responsive parenting in the first months of life was associated with later socioemotional competence. Sensitive, nurturant care is thought to be the basis of a secure attachment according to this theory (Carlson, Cicchetti, Barnett, & Braunwald, 1989). The Ainsworth et al. (1978) strange situation has been the primary instrument used for assessing individual differences in attachment patterns of children. This instrument is a laboratory-based paradigm consisting of a series of 3-minute episodes designed to activate the child's behavioral system by producing mild but increasingly stressful experiences. Children are then assigned to one of three major attachment categories based on the child's interaction and response pattern on reuniting with the caregiver during the strange situation.

The first major attachment category is known as Type A or anxious-avoidant infants. These infants display minimal amounts of affect or distress in the presence of the caregiver and an avoidance of the attachment figure under conditions that usually elicit interaction with the caregiver.

Securely attached infants (Type B) constitute the second category. These infants frequently engage in affective sharing with the caregiver and are able to seek comfort and be calmed by the caregiver when distressed.

Type C, or anxious-ambivalent, infants, demonstrate behaviors of high proximity seeking mixed with resistance to the caretaker and an inability to be comforted and calmed by the caregiver when distressed. On using this classification system, many researchers found that there was a group of infants who did not fit into any of the three classifications described.

Main and Solomon (1990) developed a new attachment pattern, Type D, disorganized/disoriented, which was not in the orignal system. Infants in this category appeared to have no apparent coping mechanism as they blended contradictory features of several strategies or appeared dazed and disoriented when reunited with their caregivers. The disorganization was characterized by a disordering of temporal sequences, incomplete or undirected movements, stilling, slow movements, freezing, depressed affect, and direct indications of apprehension toward the parent (Carlson, Cicchetti, Barnett, & Braunwald, 1989). The overall results of studies using this type of classification system have shown that maltreated infants are likely to be rated as insecurely attached to their caregivers in addition to showing a disorganized/disoriented attachment.

Carlson, Cicchetti, Barnett, and Braunwald (1989) suggested several explanations for these results, including: (a) the homes of maltreated children are characterized by a pattern of inconsistent care; (b) there is an element of fear that is essential in developing the disorganized/disoriented attachment and freezing, stilling, and dazing are signs of this type of attachment; and (c) infants of mothers with affective disorders, such as depression, are at increased risk for avoidant/resistant attachment relationships.

Other studies have been conducted to evaluate the relationship between attachment security and conversational skill development among lower SES maltreated and nonmaltreated toddlers (Coster, Gersten, Beeghly, & Cicchetti, 1989). Results have shown many attachment-related language differences in mother-child conversational samples. Despite the fact that the toddlers were all raised in a low SES environment, secure toddlers had a higher mean length of utterance than insecure toddlers. In addition, the secure group made more relevant contributions to the conversation and demonstrated a more diverse vocabulary. In another study, Cicchetti (1990) reported that securely attached toddlers were more likely to use "is" in their vocabulary. This finding indicated that children who are more secure and use more "is" language are better able to discuss internal states and feelings than are insecure children.

Morisset, Barnard, Greenberg, Booth, and Spieker (1990) evaluated the impact of environmental risk on toddlers' developing cognitive and linguistic skills. Their results confirmed that the impact of environmental risk on young children's development is influenced by the quality of early mother-child interaction. The authors further concluded that the quality of these experiences at 1 year of age was more predictive of the child's outcome than was family SES or social and psychological functioning. The mothers in the study, who reported a high level of depression, showed few interpersonal and social skills. In addition, mothers of lower SES were not as likely to provide infants with stimulation in terms of facilitating conversation, maintaining interaction in conversation, and providing a variety of vocabulary forms for the child to model. All of the above factors are important in understanding the language development of children in families at high risk for abuse and/or neglect.

Communicative Functioning

A letter from McCauley and Swisher appearing in the 1987 *Journal of Speech and Hearing Disorders* posed the unanswered question: "Are maltreated children at risk for speech or language impairment?" (p. 301). McCauley and Swisher reported that there is research to show that maltreated children have serious developmental problems, including deficits in social and emotional development, intellectual development, and language and speech skills. Research findings also support a strong independent relationship between neglect and receptive language performance and between neglect and expressive language performance.

In a follow-up study of traumatized children, Elmer (1977) matched children traumatized by abuse to children traumatized by accident. She concluded that, although no major differences existed between the groups, a large percentage of the children in the abused group exhibited language difficulties. These deficits were noted in poor articulation, expressive/receptive language, stuttering, and intermittent aphonia. The latter is of considerable interest because it may be related to tension and anxiety. Elmer also reported that many of the children evidenced depression, sadness, and anxiety. This fact is also of particular interest because many studies have reported the overtones of emotional stress and mood disorders which are secondary to the abuse/neglect but evident in the language abilities of the child.

Many of the studies evaluating the speech and language skills of maltreated children have assessed three groups of children: abused, neglected, and neglected/abused. A recent study by Culp et al. (1991) found that, although all three groups were delayed in language and speech skills, the neglected group was most highly correlated with expressive, receptive, pragmatic, and overall language delays. The three groups did not differ in cognitive development, indicating that language development is particularly at risk in an environment where there is little parent-child interaction. The authors further concluded that children who are exposed to physical and/or verbal abuse may still receive some portions of social interaction because the incidents of abuse occur in a sporadic nature. Neglect, on the other hand, is more pervasive. In this type of environment, a child does not receive the important social interaction that is critical in early pragmatic and linguistic growth (Coster & Cicchetti, 1993).

It is clear that any type of maltreatment creates interactions that are not supportive of building strong social communication skills. The abused child often experiences interactions that are hostile, overcontrolling, and inconsistent in nature. The child who is neglected may become increasingly passive as he or she is unable to use the cause-effect relationship of language for the purpose of control of the environment (Coster & Cicchetti, 1993).

The majority of the studies evaluating maltreated children have identified the vulnerability of language development in this population (Coster, et al., 1989; Coster & Cicchetti, 1993; Crittendon, 1989; Fox, Long, & Langlois, 1988; Mash et al., 1983). The consequences of the diminished ability for early socialization will affect all domains of language development. These consequences include:

1. A significantly shorter mean length of utterance (Coster et al., 1989).
2. A more limited expressive vocabulary.
3. The use of fewer references to persons or events outside the immediate context.
4. Inability to maintain conversational discourse.
5. An inability to use language to express feelings and needs (Santostefano, 1978).
6. Insufficient development of appropriate pragmatic skills.
7. Inability to use basic functional vocabulary.
8. Inappropriate social skills leading to poor interpersonal relationships with peers (Lynch & Cicchetti, 1991).
9. Difficulty in maintaining cause-effect relationships in narratives (Kemper & Edwards, 1986).
10. Inability to use abstract language effectively.

Children who have been maltreated may exhibit any or all of the above speech and language characteristics. Although all are deficits that affect communication, the difficulties with pragmatics, social skills, and the inability to express feelings and needs effectively may indicate a secondary disorder of mood and/or emotional disturbances.

Kemper and Edwards (1986) reported that stories told by emotionally disabled children resemble stories told by children at a younger age. They omit many mental states as well as "causal links for initiation and motivation" (p. 18). The authors concluded that children who are emotionally handicapped may not be able to talk about emotional states because they do not have the necessary language to do so. As a result, their narratives are hard to comprehend because the characters' actions are not linked with an intentional mental state.

It is important to identify the coexistence of a secondary psychiatric disorder in children who are maltreated. Certainly, children who are maltreated are at risk for this type of diagnosis. Warren (1992) reported that some of the signs to watch for include a history or suspicion of physical or sexual abuse and/or neglect, history of exposure to drugs in utero, and a history of attachment problems. In addition, he reported several types of psychiatric diagnoses that are associated with communication handicaps. These diagnoses include emotional disorders (overanxious, separation anxiety, adjustment, posttraumatic stress, and sundry emotional disorders), mood disorders (depressive, manic, bipolar, mixed disorders), and parent-child, family psychological stress (parent-child problem, family circumstances, psycho-social stress problems). Overall, language impairments existed in 67% of the children studied with 75% of males and 57% of females having these impairments.

Because a large number of neglected and abused children may have a coexisting psychiatric disorder, it is important to briefly define various profiles of communication for children at risk. Beetz, Galla, and Condon (1992) outlined various communication profiles including disorders of mood. They identified problem areas at the discourse level as including:

1. Paucity of information.
2. Stories are shorter with fewer complete episodes.

3. Narrative lacking in detail and embellishment.
4. Internal responses frequently not included.
5. Actions generally causally related and sequential.
6. Content is typically violent and destructive.
7. Obstacles frequently included in narrative with great frequency.
8. Little goal-directed behavior by characters.
9. Does not request more information about topics.
10. Does not vary topics.
11. Delays before responding.
12. Does not often read nonverbal cues and displays inappropriate intonational contour. (p. 3)

As an advocate for the child who has been maltreated, the speech-language pathologist (SLP) acts as a source of information for other professionals and parents to aid in their understanding of the child, for example, that he or she may not be exhibiting oppositional behavior in the classroom, but may not have the necessary communication skills to interact with others effectively. In the same respect, the child who is not communicating effectively at a conversational level may be demonstrating characteristics of a secondary psychiatric problem such as mood disorder. The literature certainly documents the prevalence of behavior problems, depression, decreased motivation, and readiness to learn in children who have been maltreated. For all of these reasons, a thorough language evaluation should be a part of the educational and/or psychological assessment of children with a history of maltreatment.

Assessment

An in-depth speech and language assessment is a crucial part of a broader multidisciplinary assessment of the child and the family unit. At a minimum, the assessment should include the areas of receptive and expressive vocabulary, syntax, abstract language, auditory language processing, speech (articulation, fluency, voice, prosody), an oral peripheral examination, and evaluation of the presence of thought disorders, emotional, and mood disorders when indicated. Although evaluation of the linguistic aspects of the child's language is necessary, assessment of the pragmatic and narrative functions of the maltreated child is of paramount importance.

It is evident from the research that the ability to utilize language in connected discourse to convey a variety of thoughts and ideas is directly related to the environment in which the child is reared. The child who grows up in an environment where there is little stimulation and encouragement to express ideas or feelings is likely to have difficulty using verbal problem-solving methods or conversational discourse skills.

Evaluation of Narrative Functioning

Narrative functioning is based on the fact that underlying any narrative is an event chain. The event chain "is a sequence of causally and temporally ordered actions, physical states, and mental states that explains what happens, why it occurred, and what consequences resulted" (Kemper & Edwards, 1986, p. 13). The actions, physical states, and mental states are the types of events that are causally linked as initiations, continuations, and resultants to form the chain event, or the narrative (Kemper & Edwards, 1986). In order to tell a story (or a narrative), the child must have the skills to relate the chain of events to explain cause and effect, or what happened and why. From this chain of events scripts develop. Scripts are causally and temporally ordered sequences, originating from activities that are regular in the child's environment, for example, birthday parties. The script provides the framework for the shared knowledge.

Storytelling evolves from the ability to use scripts and connectives. It involves the creation of symbols, characters, and the development of cause-effect sequences. The construction of intact causal event chains is dependent on the child's experiences. The child who is neglected or abused may have a limited repertoire of experiences from which to draw. In addition, these children may be unable to express their feelings and ideas because they have never been able or encouraged to do so. As a result, their stories may be disjointed and difficult to understand because they lack the chain events of actions, physical states, and mental states. Narratives are an invaluable tool for the SLP. The information obtained from a narrative can provide information regarding communicative competence, pragmatics, and linguistic skills in addition to highlighting any secondary psychiatric conditions which may coexist. In addition, the SLP may utilize the narrative in cooperation with the psychologist or psychiatrist as a projective measure for assessing emotional functioning.

Socioemotional Assessment Issues

Prizant (1992) presented issues that should be taken into consideration when conducting a communication assessment. Some questions that should be answered during the evaluation include:

1. Does the student communicate for the full range of sociability?

2. Does communicative competence change as a function of the context of the situation, or a change in partner—adult/peer?

3. During which activities does the student demonstrate the greatest positive affect?

4. Does the student's level of arousal interfere significantly with communication?

5. Is the student able to self-regulate the emotional arousal by removing him/herself from the situation, using language to problem solve, etc.?

6. Is the student able to demonstrate abilities to mutually regulate emotional arousal by asking for help, or proposing solutions to conflicts. (p. 1)

The assessment issues presented are all important in obtaining an accurate profile of the communicative functioning of the maltreated child. Again, the speech-language evaluation is only one piece of the multidisciplinary evaluation. The child who is maltreated is unique in a testing situation because generally, he or she may not be trusting of adults. On the other hand, the child may be preoccupied with monitoring the feedback from the evaluator regarding the adequacy of his or her performance. The question remains as to whether or not the information obtained from the assessment is an accurate representation of the child's performance, or whether the pattern of response represents the child's mechanism of coping in uncertain situations (Coster & Cicchetti, 1993). This issue needs to be addressed in the assessment process by obtaining information from a variety of settings and informants.

The diagnosis of communication handicaps in psychiatric disorders is important for effective intervention to take place. Baltaxe and Simmons (1988a) outlined six ways in which the relationship between communication handicaps and psychiatric disorders can be conceptualized: (a) the communication disorder may be the only disorder present, for example, a developmental articulation disorder may exist without an additional psychiatric disorder; (b) the communication disorder may coexist with a psychiatric disorder with an unclear relationship between the two, as in the case of conduct disorder or oppositional disorder; (c) communication that is disordered may be the necessary criterion in diagnosing psychiatric disorders, as in autism and schizophrenia; (d) the communication handicap may be part of the psychiatric disorder yet is not clearly outlined in the diagnostic criteria, as in mental retardation; (e) the communication handicap and the psychiatric disorder share underlying processing deficits, as in auditory processing deficits, which are commonly associated with communication disorders but also are documented in psychiatric disorders, as in ADHD; and (f) the communication disorder may serve as the basis for diagnosing a thought disorder, whether the disorder is a content of thought disorder (relates to the semantics of what is said) or a formal thought disorder (related to the pragmatics of the communication process), both of which are criteria for the diagnosis of schizophrenia and psychosis.

Identifying and Reporting Suspected Abuse

Identifying and reporting suspected maltreatment may be an assessment issue, particularly if the SLP is the first professional to be in contact with, or develop a more personal relationship with, the child. SLPs are not considered mandated reporters of child abuse in most states, but do have an ethical responsibility to take the appropriate steps if they suspect maltreatment has occurred. The important point to realize is that one does not have to be certain that abuse or neglect occurred, just that the abuse is suspected. Of course, if the child makes a direct statement about the abuse, a child abuse report must be completed.

A report should be made to the department director or school principal who will then make contact with the local or state service agency. When filling out the report, professionals must document the case accurately and in concrete terms without providing any interpretation. If the child makes direct statements regarding the abuse, a verbatim transcription of the response is important. Parents may also be notified when a child abuse report is made. This notification should not be made if the child is faced with imminent harm. The child should also be informed if a report has been made. The information given to the child will depend on his or her age and understanding about the abuse (Berliner, 1993). Too many children are maltreated in society today. Failure to report child abuse leaves a child at risk for further undesirable consequences. As service providers to the pediatric population, it is imperative that SLPs report suspected child abuse, so that maltreated children can receive the professional intervention they need.

Recent literature regarding intervention techniques for children who are at risk for developing communication and emotional behavioral disorders has focused on both the child and his or her caregivers. Accordingly, intervention should be individualized and based on the child-caregiver interaction as well as the child's and the family's strengths and weaknesses (Sameroff & Fiese, 1990). Intervention should also occur within the context of daily routines and play situations. In these contexts, caregivers can apply facilitating techniques and observe progress in a realistic environment. In addition, intervention efforts should help caregivers to develop a responsive, child-centered style when interacting with their children. This type of style involves teaching reciprocal turn-taking and interaction, based on an appropriate developmental level for the child. Responding to the child sensitively and being nondirective in activities enable the child to develop a sense of control and build emotional attachments. The caregiver develops a sensitivity to the child's emotional status as well as the needs of the child. The goal of these techniques is to increase the caregiver's competence in facilitating communication while reducing the level of stress for both the caregiver and the child.

Intervention

Among children identified as neglected or abused, the children with communication disorders may have experienced more severe levels of maltreatment before intervention occurred (Knutson & Sullivan, 1993). A child with a communication problem presents difficulty in diagnosing the maltreatment because the child may not be able to communicate what has occurred to the evaluator. Therefore, it is difficult to confirm maltreatment of children with communication disorders, which puts the population at risk for further maltreatment. The SLP can play an important role in diagnosing and treating children with communication problems who are maltreated.

In general, the language used in the therapy setting must be appropriate for the child's developmental status. Many children with communication problems lack appropriate affective vocabulary. An important goal in therapy is to teach language to convey emotion and to role-play scenarios to express different emotional states while providing the language labels for them.

As in assessment, multidisciplinary teams provide the best way of obtaining and disseminating the wide range of information needed to plan for children who are maltreated. Many times, these children will qualify for special education services and receive school-based services. The focus of school-based services is on the educational placement and programming for the maltreated child. According to Crittendon (1989), there are four basic concepts related to the treatment of maltreated children. The children must (a) perceive their environment as one that is predictable, (b) comprehend how to influence events in the predictable environment, (c) understand how to use and interpret vocabulary dealing with feelings, and (d) possess self-control and motivation to learn.

In the classroom, maltreated children may have difficulty because their behavior may be disruptive in the classroom. In addition, these children require more "normal" types of experiences to overcome the behavioral problems they experience at home. Children who are maltreated may be using their disruptive behavior as part of an overall coping strategy (Crittendon, 1989). (A professional working with a child who has been maltreated may want to respond through sympathy, concern, and expressing a desire to help.) Many times, the professional becomes more lenient behaviorally toward the child. The maltreated child may become confused by the inconsistency in the therapist's behavior and become less trusting of adults in his or her environment.

The literature shows that early intervention in the preschool years is the critical period for children to develop positive, trusting relationships with adults and peers that will later transform to positive coping strategies. The preschool teacher and other professionals will act as the most influential role models for maltreated children. Teachers of these children need to discipline in a firm but neutral manner while emphasizing the social benefits of exhibiting appropriate behavior. Children who are maltreated have difficulty labeling emotions and feelings in themselves and others. In preschool, they need to learn to recognize and understand their own feelings of anger or sadness. They also need to learn that all adults are not like their parents and can be trusted. This trust is best developed by establishing a consistent relationship with adults in the environment for both discipline and positive reinforcement.

Children who are abused and neglected often have a relationship with their parents consisting of fear and anxiety. For this group of children, it is important to prevent the need for punishment whenever possible. Discipline, when needed, should be predictable, brief, and mild. Children who are neglected are not responsive to adults at all times. Because they have many language and cognitive deficits, it is best for discipline to be minimal until they are able to understand cause-effect relationships (Crittendon, 1989).

Regardless of the type of abuse, all children who have been maltreated have in common an unpredictable and/or uncontrollable environment. Living in this type of environment has had a negative effect on both their socioemotional and intellectual development which in turn affects the course of their future development. The predictability of the people and the environment protects these children from fear and anxiety and allows them to grow in social and academic areas. This type of environment can positively influence the child's ability to learn socially appropriate ways of achieving goals. In addition, these children need to be encouraged to communicate openly and trustingly and to develop the appropriate cognitive and language skills for their ages and ability levels (Crittendon, 1989).

Development of appropriate pragmatic skills is essential in shaping self-control and prosocial skills. Children who are maltreated have difficulty initiating and maintaining conversation with adults and peers. Frequently, if the child is able to interact more appropriately, teaching him or her a nicer way to talk to people will improve the child's interactions. These positive interactions will lead to an increase in self-confidence which is essential to a positive educational experience.

Finally, if at all possible, parents should be included in the therapeutic process. Family intervention by a psychologist or psychiatrist should be recommended at the multidisciplinary evaluation/planning meeting. In cases of abuse and abuse or neglect, parents often are not cognizant of the developmental milestones that are appropriate for a child's ability level. It is necessary to educate parents, for example, that the child is not sticking his or her tongue out to be disrespectful, or that the child is not ignoring the parent's request to stop, but simply does not have the comprehension level to carry out the command. In many states, parents are offered services before the child is removed from the home. For this reason, the SLP and other professionals involved with these children should be training and educating parents as much as possible about speech-language and normal developmental milestones as well as providing hands-on training to teach parents how to stimulate appropriate pragmatic skills.

Summary

Children who are maltreated are at high risk for communication problems in all areas as a result of the environment in which they live. Although we may not be able to change the child's living environment, as professionals we have the ability to provide early intervention with both the children and their families. This intervention is critical in the areas of pragmatics, prosocialization, and discourse skills. The key to working with these children is to provide a positive, trusting, consistent environment that will foster the development of self-confidence and self-control, both of which are essential to a productive educational experience.

CHAPTER 6

Children with a History of Prenatal Drug Exposure

Definition

Drug and alcohol abuse is a problem with a long history in our society. In the last few years, the incidence of drug abuse among women of childbearing age has increased rapidly. Children who are the result of pregnancies with drug use have grown in numbers and are more noticed by the public at large as their stories are being told in the popular press. Most recently, the plight of infants born exposed to crack cocaine has heightened our awareness of the frustrating and worrisome effects of drug abuse. Reseachers and clinical professionals are still trying to piece together the range of possible developmental, physical, emotional, and behavioral characteristics that might define the child exposed to crack cocaine. Health and education professionals are now concerned, not only about the immediate effects of drugs on birth and newborns, but also the possible long-term consequences for children's development and ability to learn as they grow.

Speech-language pathologists can expect to see children with such a prenatal history on their caseloads. In fact, the children may already be there without their drug exposure having been identified. This chapter is about who the children are and what their needs might be. Currently, they are referred to as children of prenatal drug exposure or substance abuse. The phrases do not suggest when, during gestation, one or more drugs were used, nor for what period of time, nor which ones. Some children exposed in utero to drugs have been referred to as "crack babies." Although they may have in common a prenatal exposure to crack cocaine, many women who use cocaine also use several other drugs concomitantly. It has not been possible to confidently separate the effects of each drug, interactions among drugs, their interaction with poor pre- and postnatal nutrition, or with other aspects of the pregnant user's environment. Behaviors and learning problems which have been identified as the result of drug exposure cannot be said with assurance to be the result of crack cocaine in and of itself.

Incidence and Epidemiology of Substance Abuse

Contrary to popular assumptions, recent studies have found little difference with respect to socioeconomic status in the percentage of infants born to substance-abusing mothers (MacDonald, 1992). The figure most often reported hovers around 11% to 16% of all infants born in the United States. In a population at especially high risk for illicit drug use, inner-city pregnant adolescents, the rate of use of at least one abused substance has been found to be substantially higher, perhaps as high as 50% (Crites, Fischer, McNeish-Stengel, & Siegel, 1992; Office of Substance Abuse Prevention, 1990). Estimates of the number of exposed infants born each year range from around 10 to 20 thousand. However, these are probably underestimates. The estimates come from data of births, and not all children exposed and affected by a mother's substance use during pregnancy will show difficulties during the usually short hospital stay for delivery. In fact, probably fewer than half of the infants exposed show immediate effects at birth. Some children definitely show behavioral and learning difficulties later, but we do not yet know how many. Other children who do demonstrate immediate medical problems will not be identified as having been exposed to drugs during gestation. Their medical problems are assumed to come from other factors. Further, the estimates reported are for illegal drug use. They do not include infants exposed to the use of alcohol and tobacco during gestation. Researchers have just begun to provide details of the effects of *secondary* smoke on the health of a developing fetus.

More is known about the incidence of alcohol use during pregnancy than about the use of illicit drugs. Far more children are born affected by their mothers' alcohol use than by cocaine or any of the other street drugs that have received so much attention in the last several years. The incidence rate for Fetal Alcohol Syndrome (FAS) is typically described as 1 to 6 in 1,000 live births. But those figures do not take into account children with Fetal Alcohol Effects (FAE) (see the section on Fetal Alcohol Syndrome and Fetal Alcohol Effects for defining characteristics), a group only recently coming to public attention. There are probably two to three times as many children with FAE as with FAS (Sparks, 1993). Together, FAS and FAE account for more of the cases of mental retardation that any other souce, including Down syndrome or fragile X.

The difficulties in collecting accurate data on infants exposed to drugs are enormous. Often, the figures cited rely on drug testing of the mother and/or the infant at the time of delivery. Pregnant women who use drugs early in pregnancy, then desist, would not show up in these estimates. Not all infants exposed and affected by maternal drug use show symptoms immediately. Those infants would not show up in the surveys of births and hospital discharges at birth. Not all hospitals routinely screen mothers and newborns for evidence of drug metabolites in the body. Rather, mothers or infants often are screened only if there is reason to suspect drug use. Some hospitals that do screen use only urinalysis or self-report by the mother as to her drug use during her pregnancy. One urine screen at the time of delivery only gives information about the previous few days. Drugs differ in how long they remain in a person's system and therefore how long after use they can be detected by urinalysis. For example, cocaine may be detected for about 3 days after use, whereas amphetamines may show up for 1 to 2 days, and marijuana for about 7 (MacDonald, 1992).

Obviously, many women are reticent about spontaneously offering information about their drug use, especially in light of prosecution for child abuse of women who use drugs during pregnancy in some regions of the country. Even if a woman concedes drug use during her pregnancy, she may not report the full extent nor all the drugs she used; in fact, she may not remember what she used.

Methods of testing also vary in accuracy. For example, urinalysis can be affected by something as simple as the amount of water the person recently drank. A somewhat more accurate method of finding drug metabolites in neonates is meconium analysis. It can be used to determine the presence of marijuana, amphetamines, narcotics, and cocaine. An even newer and more accurate method of drug testing is hair sample analysis. It can be done in both the mother and baby and can give some information about drug use over a period of about 3 to 4 months based on analysis at different points along the shaft of hair. This method is not in use universally, and it too has its problems in accuracy. Different colors and textures of hair retain the drug metabolites to varying degrees. Haircuts will obviously destroy some evidence as will chemical processes applied to the hair (Sparks, 1993).

Drug Use Among Women

Before the last 25 to 30 years, the use of illicit drugs was thought of more as a problem among men than among women. Smoking and drinking have been medical and social problems in our society for many more years than that. It was not known until fairly recently that alcohol and nicotine crossed the placenta and affected the developing fetus. Growing numbers of young women have begun to use a variety of drugs, including, most recently, crack cocaine and phencyclidine (PCP). To make matters worse, many of these substances are physically or psychologically addicting, so that discontinuing their use can be extremely difficult for some people and would generally mean entering a drug treatment program.

Today the use of drugs to alter one's behavioral state or mood is unfortunately common, and draws on quite a variety of substances depending on the desired effects. The way in which a drug is ingested can also vary and give different effects or alter the timing of the effects. For example, a substance ingested by mouth, rather than inhaled or injected, goes into the mother's bloodstream more slowly and crosses the placenta to reach the fetus more slowly (MacDonald, 1992).

Various kinds of drinks contain different amounts of alcohol. For example, drinking tequila administers more alcohol per drink than a wine cooler. On the other hand, a woman who drinks a lighter form of alcohol, say beer or wine, may dose her body with small amounts of alcohol over a longer period.

Cocaine is used in a number of ways and is therefore ingested in differing amounts and time frames. One widespread method of taking it is called a "primo." The method combines crack with marijuana which is then smoked (Sparks, 1993). Another method of using cocaine is to inject it, alone or with other drugs such as methadone or heroin. "Speedballing" is injecting heroin with cocaine. Injection or smoking of cocaine, while reaching the bloodstream more rapidly, requires a higher dose to get the desired psychotropic effects (Office for Substance Prevention, 1990). Therefore, the fetus receiving this drug dose may be getting more toxic levels of it than if the mother "snorts" the powdered form of cocaine. However, the drug is metabolized and cleared from the body more quickly. "Snorting" cocaine prolongs the time it is in the body and therefore may harm the fetus through the longer exposure time (MacDonald, 1992).

Drugs are often combined or taken in sequence to counteract side effects or enhance the original drug's effects. Although research is still trying to get a handle on teratogenic effects of individual drugs, it seems certain that using more than one drug raises the chances of damage to the developing fetus. Further, using two or more drugs not only stacks one risk atop another, but the substances may interact and make the risk of fetal damage more likely or more serious. Some of the most frequently used drugs and how they are generally combined follow.

The most common and widely used drugs are alcohol and tobacco. The Office for Substance Abuse Prevention reported surveys in 1990 which showed that, among women of childbearing age, perhaps as many as 30% were smoking at the time of conception and 25% of them continued to smoke while pregnant. The women least likely to quit or reduce their smoking while pregnant are the youngest and poorest. They are also the mothers who have other high-risk factors in their lives which can have an impact on their developing children.

A woman who smokes and drinks is more likely than one who does not to also use illicit drugs. Women addicted to alcohol often also use one or more among caffeine, marijuana, minor tranquilizers, sedatives, and amphetamines. Heavy users of marijuana often also smoke and drink alcohol. When they become pregnant they are more likely to reduce the amount of alcohol and nicotine they use than to reduce use of marijuana.

Since the 1980s, crack cocaine has been one of the most widely used illicit street drugs. It is relatively cheap, as illegal drugs go, and is readily available. One reseach study in a large American city found that, among pregnant substance abusers, 80% were using at least crack cocaine, often with other drugs as well (American Academy of Pediatrics, 1988). Women who use crack are likely to also ingest one or more of the following: marijuana, alcohol, nicotine, narcotics, and minor tranquilizers. PCP may be mixed with marijuana, tobacco, or herbs when it is smoked.

A woman may use drugs over a period of time and may or may not become addicted to them. If she does become addicted, she may be physically or psychologically dependent. Alcohol, narcotics (heroin, methadone, Talwin [T's], blues [pyribenzamine]), and nicotine produce the physical kind of dependence. When use of one of these drugs is stopped abruptly, physical symptoms in reaction to the lack of the drug's presence occur. Cocaine, on the other hand, is not physically addicting but is psychologically addicting. When stopped, the person has no physical symptoms from its disappearance in the body, but still strongly craves the psychological effects derived from taking it. Some drugs do not seem to be addicting, regardless of the level, frequency, or duration of use.

Even in the case of the best documented drug, alcohol, pregnant women often use additional drugs, and it is not yet known how other drugs interact with the alcohol to affect the developing fetus. Not only is the amount of alcohol that must be ingested to produce Fetal Alcohol Syndrome or Fetal Alcohol Effects still in question, it is also not known what part an additional substance might play in potentiating the likelihood that the child develops those effects.

Drug Use During Pregnancy

Before the Thalidomide-affected infants it was believed that the placenta provided a barrier between toxic substances in the mother's body and her developing fetus. It turns out that the placenta is not a barrier for many subtances, but rather a conduit. All of the drugs discussed in this chapter cross through the placenta. Most also enter breast milk as well. What is known about the short- and long-term effects of drugs on infants and children varies considerably from one drug to another. Use and abuse of the drugs themselves varies. Alcohol and cigarette smoking have been around for a long time; PCP and crack cocaine have only been on the streets for a few years. Even among drugs that have been in use a long time, there is variability in how much research has focused on the teratogenic effects during gestation. For example, research on heroin use demonstrated about 25 or so years ago that infants born to abusing mothers presented with withdrawal symptoms after delivery. But not much coverage has been given to its possible long-term effects on development and learning ability. Very little is known about how PCP affects the developing fetus, in part because the drug is often part of a constellation of several substances abused.

One difficulty in making the link between drugs ingested during pregnancy and the possible resulting disorders in behavior and learning has to do with the pattern of drug use during the pregnancy. One factor is when, during gestation, the fetus is exposed. Although many women do not stop or reduce their drug and alcohol use during pregnancy, others *will* curb their use as soon as they realize they may be pregnant. The problem is that it can take several weeks for a woman to discover her pregnancy. In the ensuing time, the fetus will have been exposed to whatever the woman ingests. For many disorders, the first several weeks after conception are critical in the fetus' development. Many women do not realize how crucial these early weeks are to the development of their child, and therefore do not realize the damage their drug use may have done to their baby.

Some drugs can cause physical changes in a woman's body that mask early signs of pregnancy. Sustained use of narcotics causes irregular menses, thus reducing the likelihood of a woman detecting her pregnancy at an early point. Relatively heavy use of tobacco or marijuana, or regular consumption of alcohol, can also disrupt regular menses, and thereby mask pregnancy in its earliest stages. Use of narcotics can cause nausea, so that a woman used to nausea from drug use would not relate it to pregnancy as she otherwise might. Use of narcotics or cocaine also can produce feelings of exhaustion, masking another early sign of pregnancy.

If a woman is addicted to one or more drugs when her pregnancy begins, she is unlikely to be able to stop using those drugs and possibly others as soon as she knows about her pregnancy. Many drugs alter motivation, cognitive skill, including problem solving, and priorities in life: in general, one's mental health. It is not uncommon, for example, for a woman using drugs heavily not to seek prenatal care for her baby. Her concerns are not focused on her child, as they might be if she were not suffering the effects of drug use.

Women who are not addicted but continue to use drugs during pregnancy may use them routinely or on an intermittent basis. As with alcohol, there are as yet no exact guidelines as to how much drug use or what frequency of drug use will cause subsequent damage to the developing child. What is known is that the more drugs and alcohol are used, the greater the likelihood of long-term effects on the child.

There are other characteristics of drug use which seem to be important to the fetal outcome but the effects of which are not known. For example, what about the purity and potency of the drugs consumed? Both can vary considerably. PCP and heroin routinely are cut with a variety of other substances. Marijuana, on the other hand, is usually found in a pure form, but the potency of any batch can vary significantly.

The environmental characteristics surrounding the mother-to-be and her developing child also are important. Often a drug-abusing women receives little or no prenatal care. Her infant may not receive any better or more consistent care after birth. Drug-abusing woman often are malnourished themselves and live in very stressful and unstable conditions. Often, they are very young and very poor. These circumstances also negatively affect the development of the fetus or infant who experiences them. Research has shown that, despite a poor environment, in many ways a drug-exposed infant who receives adequate pre- and postnatal nutritional and medical care develops better than a child in the same circumstances without the intervention.

Thus far it looks as though some exposed children escape with no detectable impairment. Just as with FAS/FAE, the parameters of when and how much exposure can occur without impairment are not known. The characteristics that have been reported are shown in Tables 6–1 and 6–2 and discussed in the following sections. Drug exposed children may show some, all, or none of these.

Biological Impact of Substance Exposure on the Fetus

Most of the substances discussed in this chapter are lipophilic and have a low molecular weight. These characteristics allow them to cross the placenta between the mother and the developing fetus. They are toxic and capable of interferring with fetal development. Alcohol and cocaine are thought to decrease the blood supply to the fetus, thereby decreasing the nutrients and oxygen it should be receiving, as well as inhibiting the ability to carry carbon dioxide away from the fetus.

Cocaine (perhaps in concert with other drugs) appears to also constrict blood vessels in the fetus, thereby raising the risk of brain hemorrhage. Some research has found evidence of intracranial bleeding and/or atrophy in the frontal lobes and

Table 6–1. Known and hypothesized teratogenic effects on fetus and birth.

Drug	Direct Fetal Effects	Perinatal Effects
Crack cocaine	Disrupted development of fetal tissue Effects on various systems (e.g., CNS, urogenital, intestinal, extremities) *Altered action of neurotransmitters*	IUGR Low birth weight Restricted blood flow hypoxia decreased nutrition Prematurity Abruptio placentae
Tobacco (many carcinogens)	*Malformations* (e.g., cleft palate, CNS abnormalities)	Low birth weight (even from passive smoke to mother) Hypoxia Prematurity Placenta previa Abruptio placentae
Alcohol	Impairment of protein synthesis and metabolism	IUGR *Restricted blood flow* *hypoxia* *decreased nutrition* Abruptio placentae Fetal distress *Prematurity*

(continued)

Table 6–1. *continued*

Drug	Direct Fetal Effects	Perinatal Effects
Marijuana	No known effects	Hypoxia *Alone likely no effect on delivery but may in drug interaction*
Methamphetamines (Speed)	No known effects	No known effects
Narcotics	*Possible decrease in number of brain cells* Disrupted RNA Decreased thickness of Cerebral cortex Impaired neurotransmission Impaired cell growth	IUGR Small for gestational age *hypoxia* *decreased nutrition* Prematurity Abruptio placentae Fetal distress Breech birth Eclampsia Placental insufficiency Meconium staining Aspiration pneumonia Respiratory distress Hyaline membrane distress Brain hemorrhages

(continued)

Table 6–1. *continued*

Drug	Direct Fetal Effects	Perinatal Effects
PCP	No known effects	No known effects
Minor tranquilizers (Benzodiazepines)	Cleft lip and palate Malformations of the heart, arteries, and joints (Vallium® [diazepam]) *Especially combined with alcohol or tobacco* *Disrupted development of fetal tissue of CNS* (Librium®)	Low birth weight (all minor tranquilizers)
Short-acting barbiturates	Birth defects	Birth defects

Note: Hypothesized effects shown in italic type.

Table 6–2. Known and hypothesized teratogenic effects on newborns and infants.

Drug	Effects on Infants and Newborns
Crack cocaine	Disrupted sleep pattern Poor feeding Muscle tremors Increased muscle tone Transient EEG abnormalities Abnormal reflexes Abnormal movement patterns High pitched cry
Tobacco	SIDS Infant death from infections
Alcohol	Infant death Poor feeding Failure to thrive Higher rate of infections FAS FAE
Marijuana	No known effects
Metamphetamines	Poor feeding Disrupted sleep pattern

(continued)

Table 6–2. *continued*

Drug	Effects on Infants and Newborns
	Muscle tremors Increased muscle tone
Narcotics	SIDS Poor feeding Disrupted sleep pattern Muscle tremors Increased muscle tone Withdrawal symptoms
PCP	Restlessness Poor visual coordination Hyperresponsive to sound & touch Increased muscle tone Rapid state changes Unconsolable *Small head circumference during first year* *Mild neurologic deficits at least during first year*

(continued)

Table 6–2. *continued*

Drug	Effects on Infants and Newborns
Minor tranquilizers (Benzodiazepines)	Lethargy Respiratory problems (e.g., apnea) Low muscle tone Poor sucking Valium® (diazepam) late in pregnancy can cause withdrawal symptoms
Short-acting barbiturates	(Tuinal®) Withdrawal symptoms

Note: Hypothesized effects shown in italic type.

basal ganglia in the brains of some neonates prenatally exposed to coccaine. It is not yet known what the long-term behavioral and developmental effects of those damaged areas would be.

Alcohol is thought to cause fetal damage by decreasing protein synthesis and production of neurotransmitters and by interfering with cell growth and migration, as well as myelination of nerve tracts. Alcohol and other teratogenic drugs can affect a fetus regardless of when during the pregnancy they are used.

Characteristics of Children of Prenatal Substance Abuse

Problems Created for Pregnancy and Delivery

The use of drugs, alcohol, and smoking reduce a woman's chances to carry a fetus to term and have a normal delivery. Drinking alcohol or smoking during pregnancy can cause bleeding or ruptured placental membranes. Abruptio placentae and prematurity are risks increased by the use of alcohol, tobacco, cocaine, and narcotics. Narcotics also increase the risk of other pregnancy and delivery complications including eclampsia, placental insuffiency, breech birth position, brain hemorrhages, respiratory distress, hyaline membrane disease, and aspiration pneumonia. The rate of miscarriages and stillbirths increases with the use of alcohol and narcotics, and possibly of marijuana and cocaine, during pregnancy. Alcohol raises the risk of spontaneous abortion and stillbirth (Office for Substance Abuse Prevention, 1990).

The chance of fetal distress increases with use of alcohol and narcotics. Another possible outcome from smoking during pregnancy (even passive smoke from someone in the woman's environment) or using alcohol, cocaine, narcotics, or perhaps minor tranquilizers or marijuana during pregnancy is low birthweight, whether the birth is premature or not. Intrauterine Growth Retardation (IUGR) is another risk with alcohol, cocaine, or narcotics use. IUGR is the long-term result of poor nutrition to the fetus from the mother's body and inadequate transfer of oxygen and carbon dioxide between mother and fetus (Office for Substance Abuse Prevention, 1990). Babies with IUGR are born small for gestational age. Low birthweight and IUGR increase the risk of infant mortality, respiratory problems, failure to thrive, infections, and developmental delays and disorders later in the child's life.

Other Medical Problems and Physical Malformations

Exposure to alcohol in utero can cause heart defects, cleft lip and palate, joint malformations, auditory problems, vision disorders, poor development of dentition, liver and kidney problems, skeletal defects, increased propensity to upper respiratory infections (including middle ear infections), sensorineural hearing loss, and seizures (Office for Substance Abuse Prevention, 1990, Sparks,1993). Minor tranquilizers increase the risk of cleft lip and palate and malformations of the heart, arteries and joints, especially when used with tobacco or alcohol. Tobacco itself contains many carcinogens and *may* increase the risk of malformations such as cleft palate. Cocaine use has been linked to increased risk of various fetal systems, including the urogenital and intestinal systems and malformations of extremities.

Fetal Alcohol Syndrome and Fetal Alcohol Effects

The teratogenic effects of alcohol are discussed separately from those of other drugs because more information exists on alcohol-related disorders. Fetal alcohol syndrome is a group of characteristics that occurs in the domains of growth deficits (before or after birth), dysmorphic traits, and/or neurobehavioral problems. FAS occurs when a woman uses alcohol during her pregnancy. We do not know the amount of alcohol nor how long it must be used to produce these attributes in the infant. This is why it is recommended that women use no alcohol during pregnancy. Reduction or cessation of alcohol use at some point during the pregnancy probably lessens the degree of impairment to the developing child. The term FAE is used when there is a less severe expression of known alcohol-related characteristics. Often this simply means that affected children have more subtle physical indicators, but their behavioral and learning problems can be just as severe in the impact they have on their lives and that of their families. Children with FAS/FAE may have small stature, microcephaly, be thin, and have abnormal facies: short palpebral fissures, flat midface, indistinct philtrum, thin upper lip, micrognathia, low nasal bridge and short nose, epicanthal folds, various anomalies of their ears (Sparks, 1993).

FAE is often misdiagnosed or goes undiagnosed because it is not well recognized. Additionally, there may be no record of maternal alcohol use. Even if maternal alcohol use is noted in the child's birth records, if the child does not show any immediate effects, the link may be forgotten by the time the child presents with issues of development and/or behavior. Currently, getting the proper diagnosis for children, adolescents, and adults is a high priority, especially in some geographic regions where there may be a higher incidence of alcohol-related disorders. Children with FAE can experience years of difficulty in school and in the community without their disorder being diagnosed. They may be thought to be "lazy" or "unmotivated" in school. Children with FAE may be considered exceptionally "forgetful" and disorganized, exceptionally quiet, constant talkers, unpredictable in their behavior, or considered "behavior problems" in school.

Deficits Resulting from Drug Exposure in Utero

For infants who are exposed prenatally to drugs and survive beyond the neonatal period, here is what may be seen.

Cognition

Alcohol *can* lead to mental retardation in prenatally exposed infants. Some research indicates that cocaine, or cocaine in combination with other drugs, sometimes leads to retardation as well, although this is not the usual case (Sparks, 1993). With the drugs thus far studied, even when the child's intelligence falls within the normal range, problems of attention, interaction, and learning can result from prenatal exposure (Lesar, 1992). Children affected by prenatal drug exposure demonstrate poor problem solving and use unelaborated play schemes. They do a lot of repetition but little pretend or building on pretend themes. As toddlers they use toys in very simple ways, for example, picking things up, holding them briefly, then throwing or putting them down. In other words, there is little exploration, no attempt to work things themselves, or to combine an object in use with another (Howard, Beckwith, Rodning, & Kropenske, 1989). As substance-exposed children get older, they improve in their use of materials but still use them in less rich, more restricted, less imaginative ways compared to their unaffected peers (Rivers & Hedrick, 1992).

By elementary school, children with FAS/FAE, even with intelligence in the normal range, demonstrate difficulty with abstract thought, and later with abstract reasoning and other higher order thinking skills. Poor memory also continues to affect their school performance as well as daily living skills. In elementary school, children with FAS/FAE sometimes have achievement test scores that look better than expected given their intelligence test scores. At a later age, often between the sixth to eighth grades, their achievement scores level off and more closely match their intelligence scores. The child with FAS/FAE is more likely to have difficulty with math than with reading and related skills (Office for Substance Abuse Prevention, 1990; Streissguth et al., 1991).

As children with FAS/FAE get older, and even as adults, their inability to look ahead at the consequences of their behavior, use good judgment in what they do, and follow the rules of behavior and govern their own behavior appropriately persists. Just as when they were younger, they need close supervision so that they do not get themselves into trouble. Consequently, as adults, people with FAS/FAE may be incapable of living independently.

Attention and Response to the Environment

In neonates attention involves behavioral states and how the child shifts from one state to another. Infants ordinarily spend time in sleep and alert states. When alert, they are most available to stimulation during a quiet alert state, and most infants can maintain such a state over a period of time. In this state a baby attends to auditory and visual stimuli. By 1 month of age, babies can attend for a considerable length of time. Ordinarily, infants spend less time in a cry state. They typically shift from one behavioral state to another in an organized way.

Drug-exposed infants are less organized in their transitions from one state to another, and they make the shifts more abruptly. They spend more time in cry or sleep states, are very irritable, and difficult to calm. Some research has identified infants with prenatal exposure to cocaine as being the most difficult as a group to console (Chasnoff, Burns, Schnoll, & Bunns, 1985). Professionals who work with PCP-exposed infants describe *them* as the least easy to console among all drug-exposed infants (Office for Substance Abuse Prevention, 1990).

Drug-exposed infants have difficulty reaching and maintaining a state of quiet alertness so that they are available for stimulation. In fact, their heightened sensitivity to incoming stimuli causes rapid shifts from calmness to overexcitement and restlessness. From that point the infants will go into deep sleep or crying, depending on individual ways of blocking out what is for them too much stimulation.

Neonates exposed to narcotics seem to have difficulty directing their attention toward a stimulus in the first place. Those diagnosed with alcohol exposure seem unable to adequately screen incoming stimuli and do not habituate to constant environmental properties around them. Other drug-exposed newborns become overstimulated very quickly so that they have little time to observe and learn about visual and auditory stimuli in their environment before they have had too much. The interval between their levels of quiet alert and overstimulation seems short.

Drug- and alcohol-exposed neonates also can be disorganized in their patterns of sleep and feeding. Some substances, for example, alcohol or minor tranquilizers, leave the newborn with poor sucking ability so the child can be at risk for becoming "a failure to thrive" infant. The problems these infants experience in regulating their basic cycles for feeding and sleeping can persist into childhood, making the children's lives that much more erratic and making caring for them difficult.

When infants are overstimulated and need a break to reorganize, they use avoidance behaviors (e.g., turning their eyes away). If that does not remove the stimulus adequately, they eventually cry or withdraw into sleep. Infants identified as being drug-exposed go more quickly into crying or sleeping and therefore have less alert time available for interacting with others. Interventionists have noted that these infants do not seem to enjoy human contact the way most babies do. Rather, one of the primary sources of agitation for them is a human face. Whether they react by crying or avoiding contact in other ways, faces seem to be negative stimuli for at least some of the infants exposed to drugs.

Another source of discomfort and disruption for drug-exposed infants is handling. The normal activities of providing care (i.e., changing, grooming, dressing, and bathing) cause reactions of hypersensitivity and lead to negative reactions from the infant. Consequently, for some infants of substance abuse, human interactions do not provide pleasure and the infants do not try to elicit more contact with their caregivers.

Not all drug-exposed infants show these behavioral state differences to such an obvious degree. Therefore, not all are identified as having problems in infancy. For some exposed infants, irritability and disorganization do not become apparent until several weeks after birth.

Infants with FAS/FAE typically enjoy physical contact once an initial phase of irritability subsides. They enjoy cuddling with their caregivers and in general are very socially oriented. Often infants and children with FAS/FAE do not show the typical fear of strangers.

As drug-exposed infants become toddlers and are more capable in their motor skills, they may show their hypersensitivity to interpersonal contact and other parts of their environment in new ways. Some children of substance abuse look aggressive at this age. They hit, bang, or throw their toys. These behaviors may occur suddenly and without any observable reason. Just as when they were infants, these children reach the point of overstimulation quickly. Whereas in infancy they shifted abruptly and erratically from one behavioral state to another, now they present with labile emotions and responses out of proportion to the situation. Sometimes these children throw frequent, exaggerated, or prolonged temper tantrums.

Many of the children seem to have deficits in integrating sensory information. For example, a child may exhibit strong negative reactions to the close proximity of another person, especially peers or siblings. Other children may jostle or touch the drug-exposed youngster suddenly and without warning, not necessarily with any negative intent. For a drug-exposed child this is unpredictable and therefore threatening input. Children exposed to drugs in utero crave predictability.

Children prenatally affected by alcohol continue to enjoy interactions with people as they get older. They come across as friendly and gregarious. They also are thought of as fast-moving and energetic, sometimes to the point of hyperactivity and attention deficits. They tend not to stay long with any one activity. FAS/FAE children may show little impulse control and display a strong will and lack of responsiveness to rules and directions. Children with FAS/FAE may explode into significant tantrums just as other prenatally drug exposed young children do. Despite their strong interest in social interactions, their hyperactivity, impulsivity, and strong emotional reactions, as well as their craving for physical contact, can get them into trouble with peers.

Children with FAS/FAE may show little or no appropriate sense of danger and require constant supervision. At an age when most children can follow the rules of safety and behavior (e.g., being in a shopping mall with mom or on the playground at their preschool), children with FAS/FAE may not follow well-rehearsed rules or be amenable to the usual verbal negotiation between adult and child.

As toddlers, the disorganization in how they interact with their environment is still evident for some drug-exposed children. They may do a lot of wandering around rather than finding purposeful activity and staying with it for any length of time. They may be identified as easily distracted in attention, overfocused, and unable to make transitions easily. These children may seem impulsive in their behavioral style. Children with FAS/FAE may present as hyperactive as well. So, too, may children prenatally exposed to nicotine, although the relationship between a pregnant woman's smoking and her child's subsequent hyperactivity is less clear. As children exposed to drugs and alcohol grow to preschool age and beyond, they can continue to exhibit problems of distractability.

Social-Emotional Characteristics

The infant state characteristics described for children of substance abuse have a strong negative impact on the development of the maternal-infant bond. It is hard to care for a child who becomes irritable quickly and is in a state of irritability much of the time. Further, when the caregiver's face is a primary source of the child's agitation, the caregiver receives little positive affect from the child to whom she needs to become attached. The disorganization and irritability of drug-exposed infants' state can go on for many months after birth and, in fact, persist, becoming the children's typical response to the environment as they grow into preschool and school age.

Caregivers of children of substance abuse may not bring an emotionally healthy state to the infant-caregiver dyad either. The biological mother may continue drug or alcohol use after delivery of her baby. If the environmental circumstances that led to her need for psychotropic drugs persist, she is likely to continue using unless she goes into an addiction program. Continued drug use is a poor milieu in which to parent a child. Research shows that prenatally drug-exposed children who are given a more stable and appropriate home environment have a better outcome by school age (Crites, Fischer, McNeish-Stengel, & Siegel, 1992).

Sometimes children go into foster care because they are abandoned, abused, neglected, or because the mother continues to use drugs. Children who are exposed to drugs in utero may go through a succession of foster placements because, even as infants, they are so difficult to raise. Their negative responses to the environment also make it less likely they will bond well with anyone. In many regions of the country, foster care systems are overwhelmed and cannot take on all the children needing services. That means some children SLPs see for therapy may be left in home circumstances detrimental to their well-being and development.

For several interrelated reasons, then, children exposed prenatally to drugs are at risk for disordered emotional development. The irritability they may display at birth, as well as any emotional problems a drug abusing mother has, leads to inadequate bonding with an early caregiver. Later, as the child grows, he or she may continue to have only a tenuous trust of others based on experiences as an infant. Some researchers have also noted reduced tolerance for frustration in drug-exposed children. They give up on a difficult task or on solving a problem before the point nonexposed children do. This leaves them less opportunity to experience success and has an impact on exploration and experimentation with the environment. They do not easily learn persistence at a task (Lesar, 1992; Rivers et al., 1992).

As drug-exposed children reach preschool age and older, those with emotional lability continue to present with that characteristic. This sometimes includes aggression as well. Other drug-exposed children may respond to their daily environment by withdrawing rather than by striking out. Interventionists describe this group of children as having a very flat affect. Needless to say, children who are prenatally exposed to drugs can be at real risk for difficulties with peer interactions.

Motor

As neonates children exposed in utero to drugs and alcohol can be beset with tremors. These typically occur within a few days post-delivery, but can begin as late as several weeks after birth. In the case of alcohol and narcotics, tremors initially can be part of the infant's withdrawal from the drug environment in utero. However, the tremors can continue as part of the direct neurological effects of the teratogenic substances. Note that, in cases of exposure to other drugs, there are no physical addiction symptoms, but tremors are part of the neurological picture there too. Tremors can last for up to several months after birth. Several substances have also been noted to increase an infant's startle responses to stimuli. In the case of PCP exposure, the startle is in the form of gross motor movements in response to even slight touch or soft sound (Office for Substance Abuse Prevention, 1990).

In some substance-exposed neonates, muscle tone is so high that the infant appears rigid. This can be the case in exposure to crack cocaine and PCP. In exposure to minor tranquilizers, hypotonia is usually seen. Muscle tone can be so low that the neonate seems limp. Abnormal tone can be either extra high or low as a response to prenatal alcohol exposure (Office for Substance Abuse Prevention, 1990).

Abnormal muscle tone may begin several days after delivery of a drug-exposed child and can last for months or even into the toddler years. After that point it appears that tone becomes more normalized, and motor delays do not stand out in the research and observations to date, except in cases of alcohol exposure. Infants exposed to cocaine can have delayed integration of primitive reflexes. All of these teratogens can cause abnormal control of body movement. Children with FAS/FAE eventually show improved gross motor skills in childhood, but fine motor problems may persist.

A number of drugs introduced into the fetal environment are known to increase risk of vision problems. Newborns exposed to marijuana in utero can show abnormal visual response to lights. PCP can cause poor visual coordination in newborns. Neonates prenatally exposed to cocaine may present with poor visual tracking ability. Infants prenatally exposed to narcotics are at greater risk for developing vision abnormalities such as strabismus (Office for Substance Abuse Prevention, 1990).

Speech, Language, and Feeding Effects

One of the most frequent effects of prenatal drug exposure is interference with the infant's normal ability to feed. In addition to being life-threatening and putting the infant at risk for failure-to-thrive, feeding issues also impede normal infant-caregiver bonding that usually takes place around feeding. Alcohol, minor tranquilizers, and speed (methamphetamines) have been linked to poor sucking ability in newborns exposed to the drugs prenatally (Office for Substance Abuse Prevention, 1990). Infants exposed in utero to alcohol or cocaine (and possibly other drugs) have such long-lasting difficulties in feeding that long-term tube feeding is sometimes indicated. Cocaine-exposed infants often have a poor suck-swallow pattern, along with prolonged and frequent sleeping so that the baby is not readily available for the caregiver to feed. Cocaine-exposed infants also present with poor tongue stabilization and thrusting. They show lingual tremors, just as they show tremors in other body muscles when exerting effort. Some of these infants also present with gastrointestinal problems as well.

In infants prenatally addicted to narcotics, vomiting and diarrhea can be part of the withdrawal symptoms they experience after birth. In addition they also show many other physical symptoms of withdrawal that interfere with feeding as well as other functions, including congestion with sneezing and weeping eyes and hiccupping. Consequently, these infants are not available for a positive feeding experience. Their hypersensitivities to their environment make them further uncomfortable and unavailable. Withdrawal symptoms usually abate in about 1 month but can last for several months. Infants with FAS/FAE continue to have feeding difficulties which can last into childhood because their disinterest in food persists. Achieving milestones, such as shifting to solid foods, can cause further problems for them and for their caregivers.

One of the earliest indicators of possible prenatal drug or alcohol exposure in the neonate is a high pitched cry. It co-occurs with the high muscle tone and heightened reactivity in these infants. Some research has shown that neonates exposed to cocaine have subtle differences from the norm in the function of their auditory systems at brainstem level (Cone-Wesson, 1992). The effects of cocaine on auditory development are not yet known, but the concern is for the infant's later ability to process language. Other research has shown prenatally drug-exposed children 3 to 5 years of age do not discriminate among sounds as easily as unexposed children (Sparks, 1993).

Research studies on language or speech issues associated with in utero drug exposure have been complicated by the effects of a child's postnatal environment and how those effects interact with the original drug exposure. So far some studies have shown that improving the quality of the environment in which the child is raised can alter, at least in part, the prenatal teratogens' effects.

As toddlers, some children exposed to cocaine have been found to have delayed or limited use of language. Their purposes for using language are limited to utilitarian utterances of denial and requests. Eye contact has been found to be poor. Other studies have noted that in utero substance-exposed toddlers demonstrate delayed articulation. Heroin, in particular, has more often been linked to later problems with articulation and language (Office for Substance Abuse Prevention, 1990). Children exposed to heroin were delayed in developing beyond the early phonologic processes, for example, syllable reduction. They used a limited variety of sounds in their speech, also used gestures inappropriately, and were delayed in combining the use of speech with gestures.

Children with FAS/FAE may present with delays in the age at which they begin using words and combining them. Because many of the children are sociable and voluble, their families do not see them as language impaired. However, their expressive language can be echolalic and perseverative. As they get older, many children with FAS/FAE have a mean length of utterance that is low for their age. Early on, expressive language, when assessed, seems more disordered than receptive language, but many of the children have difficulty processing language, as well as having poor memory (Sparks, 1993). Therefore, one manifestation often reported is difficulty following directions, even in children with normal intelligence. Children with FAS/FAE also are more likely to have articulation disorders as young children. They often have dental malocclusions and micrognathia, as well as a higher rate of laryngeal and lingual dysfunctions.

At preschool age, children exposed prenatally to drugs other than alcohol are at risk for showing deficits in word retrieval and vocabulary. Poor ability with the receptive and expressive use of concepts also has been noted. Sometimes this group of children has been found to have poor expressive organization and lower than expected mean length of utterance for their age. Poor eye contact with others continues to be an issue. Many of the children use language less often than their peers, but increased volubility has also been noted (Rivers & Hedrick, 1992).

At elementary school age, children prenatally exposed to alcohol continue to present with disordered expressive and receptive language, but these disorders are often masked by the child's volubility and frequent use of questioning as a conversational strategy. Topic perseveration may also be present. Children with FAS/FAE often have poor understanding of social cues and therefore may choose conversational topics inappropriate for the situation. As the children get older, any articulation disorders that were present can generally be resolved. However, oral-facial abnormalities, when present, may continue to interfere with intelligibility.

In the early elementary school years, any language disorder continues for the children prenatally exposed to drugs. This may include vocabulary, concepts, multiple meanings of words, syntax, and verbal elaboration. However, improvement is seen in these areas, and the children improve their conversational skills with intervention over time. Articulation disorders remain at a higher than normal rate. We do not yet have clear evidence of how much of a role inadequate environment plays in the language and speech disorders. One way environment and drug exposure interact is in the problems of bonding with the caregiver. Abnormal social interactions existed from the earliest time. Added to that situation are all the other factors of the home environment, as well as the child's nutrition before and after birth. For children whose mothers smoked during pregnancy, research has shown some small links with later deficits in cognition, language, attention, and educational achievement.

Assessment

The importance of early diagnosis of in utero exposure to alcohol or other drugs allows professionals to predict which problems in development and learning the child and family may encounter. Some exposed children, right from birth, are going to have difficulty bonding with the caregiver, with the ability to take in and organize sensory information, and with feeding efficiently enough to allow necessary nutrition. Knowing about these and other issues ahead of time can prevent or mitigate some of their negative effects by using appropriate medical procedures and by teaching caregivers how to recognize, avoid, or intervene when something begins to go wrong.

FAS/FAE is a medical condition and its diagnosis thus should be made by a genetics clinic or others with training in dysmorphology. Information collected by school personnel concerning the child's academic performance and areas of deficit can be of benefit in making the diagnosis. Currently, many children prenatally exposed to drugs and alcohol are not diagnosed at birth and consequently are not followed as being at risk for disabilities. However, they may be put into foster or adoptive homes because of neglect or abuse. Regardless of whether the child remains with his or her biological family, behavioral issues may be the reason for initial evaluation. By this time the family can be at a loss as to how to care for a child whose behavior is so difficult to manage. An adoptive or foster family may have been told about the biological mother's drinking or drug use, but not about its possible later effects on the child's development and behavior, especially if the child presented as healthy at the time of adoption or on entering foster care.

A diagnosis gives the child's family, biological or not, a reason for disruptive behavior and any disabilities. Professionals can give the family information about possible future stumbling blocks for a child with this diagnosis so that everyone involved can prepare for them. When the biological family is involved, it is also important for any future children that the parents realize the consequences of alcohol and drug use. If the exposed child is still with the biological mother, the diagnosis may cause feelings of guilt about how her actions have affected her child. Interventionists may need to get her professional help to get past those feelings and on with parenting. Certainly, it is important for school and community staff working with the child to know something about the origin of the child's problems and future expectations as well.

Families and experts who work with children with FAS/FAE feel that having these disorders appropriately diagnosed is important in getting the children, adolescents, and adults needed school and community services (Sparks, 1993). On the other hand, for children prenatally exposed to *illicit* drugs, whether it is in a child's best interest to have that diagnosis as part of his or her records is more problematic. The kinds of disabilities seen in children prenatally exposed to drugs are not so different from the special needs of children with other disabilities. Perhaps the children identified as infants, could be referred to as "at risk." However, as more is learned about long-term effects of prenatal drug exposure, a child might benefit from having his or her exposure known so that future plans for needs could be made (Lesar, 1992; Sparks, 1993).

As noted, many children exposed to drugs in utero are not identified at the time of delivery. Even when there are problems with delivery or in the neonatal period, maternal drug use may not come to light as part of the child's prenatal history. Medical professionals should be aware of the possibility and consider it for any child. Drugs should also be suspected when a woman presents at a hospital for delivery with little or no prenatal care, a history of sexually transmitted diseases, or having older children who do not live in her home, even though she shows no sign of drug use.

Obtaining a history of drug and alcohol use can be problematic for professionals. Most people, even users, think of substance use as something negative and not to be talked about openly. In taking a history, the best way to get the information sought is with nonjudgmental and very straightforward questions. Questions should be very specific as well. Sparks (1993) in *Children of Prenatal Substance Abuse* recommends asking questions such as the following:

> How much have you smoked during your pregnancy? (p. 25)
>
> How much have you drunk? as well as Which drugs have you used? (p. 96)

and further questions about how much and when each substance was used.

Instruments such as the *Neonatal Behavior Assessment Scale* (Brazelton, 1984) can be used to assess infant characteristics such as behavioral state and alertness. Questions to the caregiver can give information on the baby's usual behavioral state, ability to handle various situations, and to self-organize for feeding and sleep. Observations of the caregiver with the child provide some sense of how well bonding is occurring.

As drug-exposed infants get older, they should be followed by a team of professionals with expertise in social-emotional growth, cognition (including an understanding of executive function), attention and behavior, speech, language, and oral sensory and motor development, gross and fine motor growth, and sensory integration. A team of professionals should be used for assessment as soon as drug exposure is suspected or known so that all areas of the child's development are monitored. In the event that no problems are detected at an early age, any child suspected of being substance exposed prenatally should still be assessed periodically by the team for problems that may arise at later ages.

Educators and allied health professionals should be aware of the features of FAS/FAE and drug exposure as far as we know them to this point. They should know what to expect in an exposed child in infancy, as the child grows through childhood into adolescence, and even what is known about exposed people in adulthood. All professionals need to be ready to recognize possible exposure in the case of any client or patient presenting for evaluation of any possible disability. Very specific questions regarding use of alcohol and other drugs during pregnancy should be part of *any* history taken and should be obtained on all clients coming for evaluation.

For any child of toddler age or older, who shows some behavioral problems or inadequate development and learning, it is important to observe the child at home or in the school or daycare setting. If the child has not been diagnosed as prenatally drug exposed, it should be considered as a possibility, and attempts made to rule it out. Some children with a history of prenatal drug exposure perform well on formal measures because the tasks and the examiner set the organizational framework. The same child's ability to function may deteriorate in situations with less outside structure in which the child must explore the possibilities, decide on something to do, set it up, and carry out the intention. The child has to do all these things while taking the social interactions involved into account as well.

Treatment

Infancy

The basic treatment goal for an infant who shows the neurological effects of prenatal exposure to drugs is development of a satisfactory infant-caregiver interaction. The caregiver learns how to interact with the baby so that the infant can learn to be calm and relaxed and take in stimulation in a more organized manner. The eventual goal is to increase the infant's ability to achieve some control of his or her own behavioral state. This will mean approaching the infant in ways that avoid overstimulation and resulting unavailability, learning what to do when the baby *is* overstimulated, and learning to read the child's cues as to how calm and how available he or she is. The accompanying goal is to help the caregiver be as successful as possible in her role. The aim is successful bonding between the infant and adult and helping the caregiver set realistic goals for herself and her child.

Caregivers can be taught to keep stimulation to a minimum for their infants. They will need to avoid excessive, sudden, or irregular movements and be gentle in handling. A drug-exposed baby's world needs to be very carefully structured and full of routine so that the child has a chance to internalize some regulation of his or her own. This is not an infant who can be held and socialized with by several people easily. Successful interaction with the child takes special knowledge and the ability to accurately read the cues as to the infant's internal state. Social interactions should proceed from one modality (i.e., into the line of vision, or talking to the baby first before coming near, or providing firm touch before showing one's face or talking). Then the second and finally third modality can be added.

Individual infants may show any number of distress signals and the caregiver will need to learn to read the ones coming from her child, accept that the child is having difficulty, and be prepared to respect the child's needs. If the child is not available, she should try again later with whatever she needed to do with the baby. Signs of distress can include gaze aversion, sneezing, yawning, hiccoughing, grunting, facial expressions, an increase in movement, dropping off into sleep, irregular heartbeat and breathing, gagging, and vomiting.

Once the child is overstimulated, or to avoid reaching that point, there are calming techniques the caregiver should learn to use. They include swaddling the baby in a blanket with hands at midline, using a pacifier, and rocking vertically for appropriate vestibular stimulation. Touch should be firm, slow, and gradual, especially around the baby's face, in the mouth, and on hands and feet, to reduce hypersensitivity. As a last resort, some drug-exposed infants require light sedation to decrease their irritability and allow them to rest and feed more easily.

Programs designed for drug-exposed infants and their caregivers have provided both direct developmental stimulation and any therapeutic intervention the individual child needs. For example, many infants with high muscle tone need special positioning techniques, such as sidelying, to decrease their abnormal tone. Parents are also given information from specialists (e.g., not to use jumpers and walkers, or encourage supported standing for their infants). These programs pair direct intervention with the child with parent training. The model most often used is parent-child play groups. Staff in these programs have to be mindful of the fragility of the caregiver-infant bond, the child's need for order, and the emotional health of the caregiver. It is also critical to attend to the family's other needs by working in cooperation with other community resources such as drug-treatment programs, job training services, counseling, literacy, and GED programs.

Infants exposed in utero to drugs and alcohol often show a poor ability to feed adequately at or soon after birth. Many of them are also hypersensitive and hyperreactive to tactile, visual, and auditory stimuli. Because they spend more time than normal in crying and can have high muscle tone along with lots of extraneous movement from irritability, they require extra calories. These characteristics are often accompanied by poor feeding and therefore lower than normal caloric intake. The result is an infant who loses weight. Additionally, drug exposure contributes to problems in digestion of food. For a drug-exposed infant, gagging and spitting up may indicate distress or be a result of difficulty with digestion. The most conducive feeding situation teaches the caregiver how to take these factors into account. The infant may need to be held in a sitting position and in slight flexion just as one would for other infants with abnormally high tone. The baby's chin should be tucked and the caregiver may need to provide external jaw stabilization. The traditional method for infants is to place the index finger on the front of the chin and the middle finger under the baby's chin. The caregiver should be cautioned to take plenty of time with feeding and be taught to let the baby alternate between feeding and resting for as long as necessary. The caregiver must expect to provide frequent but small meals. If necessary, the caregiver may need to wake the infant for feedings at regular intervals. Feeding should take place under soothing conditions, for example, using soft lighting and calming music.

Toddlers and Older Children

A number of programs have been set up around the country specifically for children known or presumed to have been exposed to drugs prenatally. These programs offer suggestions for intervention with substance-exposed children. Although there are different emphases among the programs, substance-exposed children are just like children with different developmental histories in their need to be evaluated for strengths and needs. A plan of development and education proceeds from there. All drug-exposed children are not alike nor are they necessarily different from other special needs children. Therefore they can be taught in the same early intervention programs.

One of the most important components of a program for drug-exposed children of any age seems to be strong external structure with a heavy emphasis on established routine. Some educators have found a behavioral system to be very helpful to the functioning of the children. This can be especially useful in managing aggression, tantrums, and other out-of-control behaviors that impede social interactions and classroom learning. Other programs use at least a structure which includes as few transitions as possible. When transitions *are* made, they need to be carried out very slowly and the child prepared beforehand. The cues for the transition may be verbal, visual, auditory, or a combination.

For some children with a history of prenatal drug exposure, as with other children with disordered neurological systems, it reportedly helps to provide a learning environment that is not too stimulating. Visual and auditory stimuli need to be kept to a minimum so as not to overload hypersensitive systems. Well-defined spaces can be provided for the daily tasks that are part of the classroom routine. Toys and materials need to be put away as used, and the number of things out and spread about can be limited so that children do not become overstimulated.

Some schools have encouraged a closer teacher-child attachment for substance-exposed youngsters. A child might keep the same teacher for more than 1 year. Other programs encourage closer peer group attachments by keeping classmates grouped together from year to year. These arrangements are used to mitigate the poor social relationships some drug-exposed children have at home. They also are meant to provide additional continuity and structure for lives that may be surrounded by chaos at home.

In other schools, drug-exposed children are included in regular education classrooms. Generally, what sets them apart, if anything does, and also may lead to the initial diagnosis of prenatal substance exposure, are behavioral, attentional, and emotional difficulties that arise. Some of the children are unable to stay focused on the task at hand. In a reading group they may be attending one minute and completely distracted the next. Some experts have reported that the use of stimulant medications, typically used with other children with ADHD, is not as successful with the children of drug exposure.

Case Management

There are a number of issues to keep in mind when seeing a child exposed prenatally to drugs and alcohol. The issues revolve around the child's home life and the stressors and family situation that frequently exist and are related to the mother's drug and alcohol abuse.

Obviously, it is in the child's best interest to live in a family where drug use is not part of the milieu. One of the family goals might be getting the child's mother into drug treatment. Any child, and especially one with special needs, who is difficult to bond with and to care for, is at risk for abuse and neglect by a caregiver who is herself abusing drugs and alcohol. Even a caregiver who is in chemical recovery is in a somewhat fragile emotional state, and the risk of child abuse is higher than if drugs and alcohol were not involved. There are also data to show adverse developmental effects on children who passively receive drugs (e.g., through smoke in their environments) (Randall, 1992). If the biologial mother is breastfeeding her infant and is using drugs, she can pass most drugs on to her infant through her milk, further increasing the child's exposure at a vulnerable time in life (Sparks, 1993).

These factors make it necessary for professionals working with substance-exposed children to be prepared to use the child protective services in their community for the child's well-being. By law, professionals are obligated to report any known or suspected incident of child abuse or neglect. Working with prenatally drug-exposed children also often entails working with other agencies in the community. Although educators and allied health professionals focus on the child's best interest, that may not coincide with the focus of other agencies. One example is drug treatment programs. The focus of these programs may have more to do with the person in treatment taking responsibility for his or her own actions or inaction than with the children's needs. Treatment will involve the recovering person learning how to do the day to day things any person must get done to keep going.

It is essential for professionals who intervene with drug-exposed children to keep realistic expectations for what will be possible to do to improve their lives. Even for professionals accustomed to working with very needy families, drugs worsen living conditions. Continued parental drug and alcohol use can wreck a child's opportunity for adequate physical and emotional development. Professionals know their work generally makes a difference in the quality of life for the clients they treat. It can be stressful and frustrating to feel one may not be able to have much effect in a situation. In fact, where drugs and alcohol and other stressors such as poverty are involved, the child's situation may get worse rather than improving. Feelings of frustration can also stem from thoughts that the situation could have been prevented, unlike others that result in disabling conditions for children. Consequently, interventionists may find it difficult to have the patience required for teaching and guiding a parent who has used drugs and caused damage to her child.

Summary

Exposure to drugs and alcohol in utero can have a range of effects from minimal or nonexistent to devastating. For children who do present with effects, the result can be physical as well as preventing normal learning across most areas of development. As long as these substances are available and the factors promoting their use exist in our society, medical, educational, and therapeutic specialists will be working to attenuate their damage.

CHAPTER 7

Autism and the Pervasive Developmental Disorders

with Clyde L. Robinette, Psy.D.

Definition

Autism and pervasive developmental disorder (PDD) are developmental disorders that can run the gamut from severe to mild. They appear early in life, have an impact on the child's subsequent development and learning, and are lifelong neurologically based disorders. Children diagnosed with autism or PDD have, by definition, a constellation of characteristics and behaviors which are the basis of diagnosis.

In 1943 Leo Kanner, a child psychiatrist, described a cluster of symptoms he had observed in a number of children as early infantile autism. The syndrome was later referred to as Kanner's syndrome (Kanner, 1943). He selected the term autism because he saw withdrawal from or indifference to human social contact as the essential feature of the disorder. Early speculation about causal factors centered around two sources: cold, unnurturing "refrigerator parenting" and the early onset of schizophrenia or childhood schizophrenia. We now know that neither of these factors account for the cluster of symptoms in autism or PDD. Rather, these children have a neurological disorder with several potential underlying causes. Most experts believe there are multiple biologic sources for these disorders. One form seems to have an inherited genetic basis. A family that already has one child with autism or PDD has an increased risk of having additional children with these disorders. It appears that the genetic form can be recessive or dominant. Researchers also have found that these disorders sometimes occur in families with other disorders such as fragile X, Tourette syndrome, learning disabilities, and mental conditions such as depression or obsessive compulsive disorder.

Most children with autism and PDD require a team approach to assessment and intervention because they have disabilities or delays across several developmental areas. A speech-language pathologist (SLP) will certainly be one professional from whom a child will need a great deal of service because, by definition, social interactions and the development of useful communication are universal needs of children with autism and PDD. Clinicians who see very young children may be the first education or allied health professional to see a child with autism or PDD. The first concern for parents is often delayed development of expressive language. Once the SLP sees the child he or she may quickly recognize autism and PDD as a possible diagnosis and refer the child for further evaluation by psychologist, developmental pediatrician, or psychiatrist.

Incidence and Possible Sources

Autism and PDD are estimated to occur in about 1 in 1,000 births. However, in their milder forms, they sometimes go undiagnosed for years, and the incidence may actually be somewhat higher. Autism and PDD occur four times more often in boys than in girls and are found across cultures and races (Autism Society of America, 1991).

There is speculation that some cases of autism and PDD may be more extreme expressions of characteristics and propensities that one or both parents have. This may be especially likely when mental retardation is not associated with the autistic characteristics and when the child has some areas of higher than average ability, such as in Asperger syndrome. In other words, the features of autism and PDD are like mental retardation with respect to the normal range; it is not an either/or situation, but rather a continuum of abilities. The difference is that autism has features along several continua—social, communicative, sensory, and motor. It takes the co-occurence of several of these to form the diagnosis of autism and PDD.

Another possible source for some autism is abnormality in motor areas of the brain. The idea of a possible motor component arises from the atypical gross motor movements (unusual gait and posturing, toe walking, rocking) and smaller motor stereotypies (hand flapping, finger flicking) noted in children with autism and PDD. Some research has looked at the cerebellum as a possible site of dysfunction or abnormality. Some studies, although not all, have found abnormalities there (Courchesne, 1989). Other structures in the brain are being scrutinized at the anatomical and biochemical level (Dawson & Lewy, 1989).

A higher percentage of children with autism and PDD require augmentative communication than the population as a whole. This again suggests a motor component in the disorders. Observations arising from the use of Facilitated Communication and the need for augmented/assisted communication in general suggest dyspraxia affecting the initiation and inhibition of movement. Dyskinesia (impaired ability for voluntary movement with resulting abnormal movement) and bradykinesia (slowed initiation of movement) also may be involved.

Associated Disorders

Autism and PDD are known to be related to the onset of certain diseases or conditions the child is exposed to any time during the period of gestation up to 3 or 4 years after birth. Maternal rubella, untreated phenylketonuria (PKU), cytomegalovirus (CMV) in utero, and encephalitis are examples of diseases that have been linked to autism and PDD thus far. Fetal chemical exposure has also been found associated with the development of autism and PDD (Autism Society of America, 1991).

Although autism and PDD are completely separate from mental retardation, they often co-occur. The estimated percentage of individuals with autism and PDD who also have mental retardation is approximately 70% (Powers, 1989). Fragile X is probably the source of retardation most often associated with autism and PDD. Retardation and autism or PDD can also co-occur with Down syndrome. Both disorders can result from maternal rubella or cytomegalovirus exposure. Children with autism and PDD also are at greater risk than the general population for developing seizures, especially in adolescence when the co-occurence rate is 25%. They also are at greater risk for having significant visual or auditory impairments (Volkmar, 1989).

Diagnostic Criteria

Autism and PDD are a group of related disorders. The primary features include: (1) qualitative impairment in social interactions, (2) qualitative impairment in communication, and (3) a restricted repertoire of behaviors, activities, and interests. Most professionals use the term autism to refer to children who have the classic features of infantile autism as defined by Kanner. They use PDD to refer to children who have many of the features of the autistic disorder but to a lesser degree. Actually, pervasive developmental disorder refers to a category of disorders with autistic disorder as the prototype of the category. Other disorders are Asperger syndrome and pervasive developmental disorder not otherwise specified (PDDNOS). The categories and diagnostic criteria are defined in the *Diagnostic and Statistical Manual of Mental Disorders, Fourth Edition* (DSM-IV) published by the American Psychiatric Association (1994). The shorthand version of autism versus PDD came from the revised third edition of the DSM (DSM-IIIR) (APA, 1987). In DSM-IIIR there were two categories of Pervasive Developmental Disorders: Autistic Disorder and PDDNOS (Not Otherwise Specified) for those who did not meet the full criteria for Autistic Disorder. The recently released DSM-IV includes three new diagnostic categories under the Pervasive Developmental Disorders and includes the term Atypical Autism under the category of PDDNOS. The diagnostic criteria for Autistic Disorder listed below are from DSM-IV. The new diagnostic categories of Rett disorder, childhood disintegrative disorder, and Asperger disorder are described in less detail. However, the current chapter will continue to refer to the two shorthand categories of pervasive developmental disorders that are currently in use among most professionals, namely, autism and PDD. It will take some time for the new DSM-IV criteria to gain wide professional use and for relevant distinctions in treatment approaches to emerge.

The specific diagnostic criteria for Autistic Disorder in DSM-IV are:

A. A total of six (or more) items from (1), (2), and (3), with at least two from (1), and one each from (2) and (3):
   (1) qualitative impairments in social interaction, as manifested by at least two of the following:
      (a) marked impairment in the use of multiple nonverbal behaviors such as eye-to-eye gaze, facial expression, body postures, and gestures to regulate social interaction
      (b) failure to develop peer relationships appropriate to developmental level
      (c) a lack of spontaneous seeking to share enjoyment, interests, or achievements with other people (e.g., by a lack of showing, bringing, or pointing out objects of interest)
      (d) lack of social or emotional reciprocity
   (2) qualitative impairments in communication as manifested by at least one of the following:
      (a) delay in, or total lack of, the development of spoken language (not accompanied by an attempt to compensate through alternative modes of communication such as gestures or mime)
      (b) in individuals with adequate speech, marked impairment in the ability to initiate or sustain a conversation with others
      (c) stereotyped and repetitive use of language or idiosyncratic language
      (d) lack of varied, spontaneous make-believe play or social imitative play appropriate to developmental level
   (3) restricted repetitive and stereotyped patterns of behavior, interests, and activities, as manifested by at least one of the following:
      (a) encompassing preoccupation with one or more stereotyped and restricted patterns of interest that is abnormal either in intensity or focus
      (b) apparently inflexible adherence to specific, nonfunctional routines or rituals
      (c) stereotyped and repetitive motor mannerisms (e.g., hand or finger flapping or twisting, or complex whole-body movements)
      (d) persistent preoccupation with parts of objects

B. Delays or abnormal functioning in at least one of the following areas, with onset prior to age 3 years: (1) social interaction, (2) language as used in social communication, or (3) symbolic or imaginative play.
C. The disturbance is not better accounted for by Rett's Disorder or Childhood Disintegrative Disorder. (p. 5)

Again, the diagnostic criteria for autistic disorder serve as the prototype pervasive developmental disorder from which PDDNOS is derived. The term PDD (atypical autism in DSM-IV) has been used when there is a severe impairment in social interactions, communication skills, and/or stereotyped behaviors, activities, and interests, but the full criteria for autistic disorder are not met.

The new categories of pervasive developmental disorder in DSM-IV include *Rett disorder*, childhood disintegrative disorder and Asperger disorder. Rett disorder includes a pattern of normal development through the first 6 months. Between 6 months and 4 years of age, there is the onset of decelerated head growth, development of stereotyped hand movements, loss of social engagement, poor coordination, severe language delays, and psychomotor retardation. The disorder is found only in females. Because the disorder is so pervasive and severe to profound retardation is typical, it is associated with the more severe autistic disorder.

Childhood disintegrative disorder is characterized by normal development through the first 2 years then a significant loss of previously acquired skills in the areas of social interaction and communication and the development of stereotyped patterns of behavior, activities, and interests.

Asperger disorder is a milder form of pervasive developmental disorder, often referred to as "high functioning autism." There is no delay in receptive and expressive language, cognitive development, or adaptive behaviors. The disorder is characterized by an impairment in social functioning (poor eye contact, lack of social reciprocity and initiation of interaction with others) and repetitive and stereotyped patterns of behavior and interests (obsessive interest with certain topics, inflexible adherence to routines or rituals, and repetitive motor mannerisms). Asperger disorder is often identified much later than other pervasive developmental disorders, often in middle childhood to adolescence. Some people are not identified until adulthood when their own children are being diagnosed with a pervasive developmental disorder.

To further complicate the diagnostic picture, the category of "autism" was added as a disabling condition in the regulations implementing the Individuals with Disabilities Act (IDEA) (*Federal Register*, 1992). The criteria for the educational category is as follows:

> "Autism" means a developmental disability significantly affecting verbal and non-verbal communication and social interaction, generally evident before age 3, that adversely affects a child's educational performance. Other characteristics often associated with autism are engagement in repetitive activities and stereotyped movements, resistance to environmental change or change in daily routines, and unusual responses to sensory experiences. The term does not apply if a child's educational performance is adversely affected primarily because the child has a serious emotional disturbance (p. 5)

The category of "autism" as an educational disabling condition was felt to be sufficiently broad to include the other pervasive developmental disorders. To determine an educational disability and eligibility for special education services, it is not necessary to know all of the differential diagnostic criteria in DSM-IV. However, that information may be useful in making placement decisions and IEP development.

Characteristics of Children with Autism and PDD

Social and Communication Characteristics

Any one individual with the disorder of autism or PDD will not show all of the behaviors called "autistic," and children with other disorders are sometimes referred to as having "autistic-like behaviors." The numerous characteristics and behaviors that can be shown by children with autism or PDD follow.

Symbolic behavior in general seems to elude individuals with autism and PDD (Prizant & Wetherby, 1989). Their disordered language is one aspect of their difficulty with symbolic behavior. Their understanding of the world and of language is so concrete as to make accomodation to symbols beyond their comprehension. They learn which words are to be said given a situation, and always say those words in that situation. A concrete outlook is expected from people with retardation, but even for those with autism and PDD but no retardation, the symbolic nature of language remains elusive.

This concrete focus is seen clearly in the play of children with autism and PDD. They do not exactly ***play*** with toys. Nor do they explore new ways to use a toy. In fact, in attempting to maintain order in their surroundings, they generally do not ***want*** a new activity for a familiar object. Children with autism or PDD use toys in a process of putting things in order or making things happen in routine ways so that all seems right to them. Clinicians may recognize this as the child who becomes infuriated if train cars come unhitched. Another example is tantruming when someone puts a toy figure in a toy bus for a ride when the child usually moves the bus around empty. Such a small change in routine is devastating for that child.

In contrast, many children with autism or PDD are much better at constructive play, which is very concrete and can be done in a very routine way, which must make it comforting for them. Symbolic, representational play can be combined with construction, but generally is not by children with autism or PDD. For example, a 5-year-old child with a language disorder but not autism or PDD builds large but simple structures which then become the stage for elaborate play scenes with characters from favorite television shows. A 5-year-old with PDD builds elaborate, detailed structures but has no pretend play at all to go along with them.

One of the most striking characteristics of young children with autism or PDD is the paucity of their verbal and nonverbal social interaction with others. The children appear unrelated, disconnected to, and sometimes disinterested in, others around them. Without intervention they will withdraw into their own world, where presumably they can provide themselves with some order or regularity amid what they perceive as chaos. Often parents initially view their nonresponsiveness as a hearing loss and worry that their child may be deaf. Then, once they see the child respond to quieter sounds, they begin to think of the child as "stubborn," "having a mind of his or her own," or "choosing not to pay attention." This can be devastating to parents who may feel that their child does not love them or want to be with them.

Children with autism or PDD may or may not look less at others around them. For some children, it is how and when they use social eye contact that feels different to those around them. Lack of facial expression, body orientation away from others, and not focusing directly on people when talking contribute to the impression of inattention to others. Children like this are attending to people although they may not always make sense of what they see in faces and hear from others. Children with autism or PDD **do** attend, because they learn to do new things from observing others (Bauman, 1993).

With appropriate intervention, children can begin to learn about facing others to talk and listen, approaching others, and additional conventions of conversation. However, for many children with autism or PDD, the quality of interactions will continue to be mechanical. For example, imagine the 8-year-old who wanted to share some news. Watching him come over to stand in front of the adult gave the impression of a child running onto a stage, standing straight and with his arms stiffly to his sides, squarely facing the audience to deliver his lines: "I'm coming to my friend's house to play basketball with him today."

Many descriptions have portrayed the child with autism or PDD as avoiding all social or physical contact. Although some children with autism or PDD avoid contact in the extreme, most do seek comfort from parents, grandparents, and other caregivers with whom the child is very familiar. However, the contact often must be initiated by the child. Other than providing comfort, the children may seek out others only for the intent of making requests. They may use an adult to participate in a routine activity, get something to eat, or do something the child cannot do for him- or herself. In other words, such children use language to control another's behavior to get specific needs met. It is this type of interaction that has been described as "using people like objects" in contrast to the more social use of communication called joint attention where the adult and child share an experience and enjoy each other's company.

Insights have been gained into the experience of autism and PDD from older children and adults who have developed language and have shared their perceptions. They report that social interactions and communication from others are very confusing and seem to change constantly (Grandin & Scariano, 1986). It is not that people with autism and PDD are not interested in social interactions, but rather that they avoid them because of this unpredictability. Because children with autism and PDD are unable to make sense of and sort out the intentions of the behaviors others use toward them (verbal, gestural, facial, prosodic), they are unable to use these interactive behaviors as models. Therefore they cannot appropriate these behaviors for their own use with others as normally developing children do. Higher functioning persons with autism or PDD describe developing social skills through memorizing rules for social situations and appropriate responses. They learn to follow the rules without understanding why people behave as they do.

Young children with autism or PDD develop very idiosyncratic ways of expressing basic meanings. As a result, their behavior is incomprehensible to most people. Parents often become critical mediators between their children and the rest of the world. For example, consider the 6-year-old who chants "elephant, elephant" when he wants to watch his Aladdin video. His parents may be the only ones who know that his favorite part of the movie was an elephant who had an insignificant part. Another example is the 7-year-old who shouts "Amtrak" when she feels anxious. The use of that word to express that feeling might be traced to her having heard that word at another time when she was feeling anxious. This example also demonstrates how closely tied an experience and the language during it are for children with autism and PDD.

Echolalia is often a feature of the language of a child with autism or PDD, if the child develops spoken language. It may be that echolalia is the result of a group of characteristics, some being things the child does easily, and some being weak areas of development. For example, although children with autism or PDD do not process language well semantically, they often seem to have good auditory memory. The combination of these two characteristics means that auditory memory may be used in some unusual ways (e.g., verbatim recall of long story passages, television commercials, and songs).

Echolalia can have different functions for different children and may serve several functions for one child. For example, it is often used as an affirmation instead of saying *yes* (most children use echolalia this way before they learn to use *yes*). Echolalia may be used when a child realizes he or she is expected to say something, but does not know what, or cannot formulate it. The child with autism and PDD may enter the classroom each day repeating a television commercial as a way of saying "Hi, I'm here!" Echolalia also may represent a child's attempt at comprehension through reauditorizing a message, a way of playing it back for a second chance to hear it. It also may be used as a rehearsal strategy for new information. A child may use echolalia as a way of recalling a pleasant memory. Children may also use echolalia to block out speech or other sounds or as a means of escaping from a nonpreferred activity. For example, they may repeat something with extra intensity when they are overwhelmed by external stimulation or when they do not want to do the activity being presented.

A language characteristic of children with autism and PDD related to echolalia is that they tend to be gestalt (or chunk) learners of language. Many children with autism and PDD develop language skills beyond echolalia, and they tend to learn them through a gestalt approach. The size of the chunks learned can vary from single word responses to complex language. As gestalt learners, children with autism or PDD learn language as part of a whole situation, (get meaning from the language and some of the parts), then recombine them to make novel utterances (Prizant & Wetherby, 1989). However, because of the difficulty they have in making sense of social and language interactions, the specific meanings they infer from the interactions and the recombinations of language concepts they make can be idiosyncratic. The phenomenon of pronominal reversal is related to the gestalt language learning process. The children learn a phrase that has been used toward them in a situation and echo back the phrase as their own communication. For example, if the child has always been asked, "Do you want fish crackers?" he or she may request them by asking the same question in exactly the same form without changing the pronoun.

Voice and Prosody

When a child with autism or PDD begins speaking, very often we find unusual characteristics of both voice and rhythm. The loudness level may be aberrant with no apparent recognition on the child's part that he or she is speaking more softly or loudly than others. Using a voice appropriate for the classroom, for inside, or other specific places may need to be goals for intervention.

Rhythm and rate also are commonly affected by autism and PDD. Most often, children will sound monotonic. On the other hand, they may use exactly the same inflection originally heard as part of the gestalt of the utterance. Children may use the same inflection each time they say those words, no matter what the situation. Grasping the rules of the suprasegmental features of speech is difficult for them. This can be observed even in a child who is musically talented or one who recognizes birds by their calls and songs (i.e., with auditory systems other than speech).

Behavioral Characteristics

Another major area of of dysfunction in children with autism and PDD is their restricted repertoire of behaviors, interests, and activities. Often these children have certain behaviors, topics, or actions on which they tend to perseverate. For higher functioning children, the perseveration may be on a certain topic, such as elevators or airplanes. Children with PDD may cling to a certain book with pictures of airplanes, constantly flipping through the pages and commenting. The children may approach any adult and talk about riding on an elevator, always using the same words and describing the same events over and over. Other children may have a certain repetitive way of playing with toys. They may always line them up, no matter what the toy, or they may only select toys with wheels and repetitively spin the wheels. Some children develop a behavior of moving things past their eyes in a horizontal plane. They may do this with an object at eye level on a table or windowsill. Alternatively, they may lie on the floor and move the toy back and forth. Children with greater impairment may have a particular behavior in which they will engage repetitively when there is no competing activity. In its milder form it may include rocking or stereotyped movements, such as hand flapping or finger flicking. In the extreme, the repetitive behavior can include self-injurious behaviors. These can be head banging, pulling out hair (trichotillomania), biting, and picking, pinching, or scratching their skin, all to the point of physically hurting themselves.

A related phenomenon for children with autism and PDD is a compulsive insistence on sameness in their environment. These children may become extremely upset if a chair is moved from its usual place or if the class goes outside instead of to the usual table activity after greeting/circle time.

Management of these behaviors in children with autism and PDD can be difficult because of the self-stimulatory and self-regulatory nature of the behaviors. Some children react strongly to attempts to stop or redirect them from these behaviors, with reactions that range from escalating the behavior, to screaming tantrums, to aggressive behavior toward the person who is trying to stop or redirect them. They may use the repetitive, undirected, self-stimulatory behaviors as a way to feel calm and in control of themselves. They may be trying to impose order into situations which feel confusing or uncertain because they are unable to process information that would give meaning to events around them. Higher functioning individuals with autism have reported that these repetitive activities serve to organize their sensory experiences and bring them some sense of control over what they perceive as a confusing, overwhelming array of sensory information.

Sensory Characteristics

The neurological functioning of children with autism and PDD affects their interpretation of the world around them. They often have sensory and perceptual systems that distort incoming information as opposed to delayed development of these systems. As a result they react to sensory information in unusual ways and may seek out certain types of sensory information more than other children. Some children with autism or PDD develop sensory compulsions, routinely touching , smelling , tasting, or visually examining everything before using it. The exploration of things through their senses is often an intense process that may occur quickly or over an extended period of time. For example, unless you are watching closely you may miss seeing that one child quickly puts everything to his nose before using it. Another child may spend hours, if permitted, exploring the effects of light through his moving fingers.

A second sensory characteristic is that some children with autism and PDD react strongly and inconsistently to sensory input. Some children may be hypersensitive to some stimulation and others hyposensitive. Clinicians may see both hyper- and hyposensitivity in the same individual and within the same sensory system. For example, a child may not seem to notice a sibling in the same room banging the piano keys but may become extremely upset over the sound of a telephone ringing or the short ding of a kitchen timer. Some children may seek out a certain sound or visual stimulus, but react strongly when someone else is in control of when the stimulus starts, the intensity, and when it ends.

Certain patterns have been observed in the responses of children with autism or PDD to sensory input. One of the more commonly noted is the child's response to visual information. Children with autism and PDD often avoid eye contact but seek intense visual exploration of many objects. They seem to be more comfortable gathering information through visual exploration of objects, looking at contours, varying intensities of light, movement, and other physical characteristics. At the same time some children prefer to explore their visual field through their peripheral vision, not necessarily as a way of averting their gaze, but rather as a preference. Auditory processing difficulties are another common factor in the sensory functioning of children with autism and PDD. As noted earlier, there may be both hypo- and hypersensitivity to sounds.

Many of these physical and sensory characteristics are indicative of underlying sensory integration difficulties in children with autism and PDD (Bauman, 1993). Several sensory systems are of concern. One of the earliest to mature is the vestibular system. This system of balance and posture provides information about movement and gravitational pull. Children with autism and PDD frequently present with behaviors and responses to their environment which indicate abnormal processing of information through the vestibular system. Clinicians may see children who cannot seem to get enough of certain types of movement. Swinging is often very important to these children. Alternatively, the child may have abnormal fear of certain kinds of, or even most, movement. A child like this may get upset when encouraged to use outdoor play equipment.

Another important and early maturing sensory system is the kinesthetic/ proprioceptive system. It provides information on touch and body position. Locations of nerve endings for this system are in the muscles, tendons, joints, and skin. When this system is functioning well, the incoming information is interpreted and guides the rest of the central nervous system, providing awareness of location of the body and its parts in space and how the body is positioned with respect to other people or objects around it.

The importance of the vestibular and kinesthetic/proprioceptive systems in concert is that they provide appropriate balance (against gravity and during movement). If a person does not have good balance reactions, he cannot have good quality of movement. He or she will feel unsafe and insecure. The two systems in concert also provide a person with a sense of being organized and knowing his place within his environment even when that environment changes. These are feelings crucial to a sense of well-being and security. Tactile information must be adequately and efficiently processed and integrated into the child's image of himself as he fits into his surroundings, both social and physical. A person's tactile system, when not working appropriately, can be hyper-reactive, hyporeactive, or alternate between the two extremes. Many children with autism and PDD frequently are hyper-reactive to several kinds of input including tactile. This condition is called tactile defensiveness. Children with tactile defensiveness may not be cuddly. A defensive reaction to touch will be elicited by a light touch from other people or objects, such as a breeze or blades of grass. It may also be manifested as a response to certain textures and temperatures. Children with tactile defensiveness may react to soap, especially on their hands. They may get upset when encouraged to fingerpaint or play with Playdoh. They may refuse to wear new pieces of clothing, and have a difficult time switching seasonal clothes when seasons change.

A person with tactile defensiveness may also be hypersensitive to incoming stimuli through the other modalities of vision, hearing, taste, and smell. This additional hypersensitivity is common in people who have autism and PDD. In fact, the poor eye contact and the purposeful gaze aversion so often observed in children with autism and PDD may be hypersensitive responses to other people. In social interactions, people do considerable moving and changing with their bodies, and especially their faces, in ways that are filled with meaning for most people. The amount and rate of changing information may be overwhelming to the processing capabilities of the person with autism and PDD. Clinically, you may observe a child with this hypersensitivity trying to block out stimulation overwhelming him or making him feel out of control. He may cover his ears, eyes, nose, or mouth; avert his eyes, or use repetitive body movements until he feels under control or the offending stimulus goes away.

Imagine being distracted or set on edge by sights, sounds, smells, or touch that are simply part of your daily environment. The same things are disregarded by most people. A child's attention, ability to learn from events, and communication are interrupted. In other words, the child with autism and PDD who is hypersensitive is missing out on important input at the same time he is feeling assaulted by what the rest of us consider inconsequential phenomena. Another result of being hypersensitive to touch can be that the child does not like the feel of objects in his hand. Clearly fine motor and visual motor skills can not develop typically if the child cannot tolerate holding handles, tools, lids, or other things long enough to learn how to work with them.

The many ways in which a child with autism or PDD is unable to adequately and accurately integrate incoming sensory information from the several modalities can cause him to feel overwhelmed. Indeed, this is how many children with autism and PDD present, as being easily overstimulated, which, depending on the child, may result in tantrums, repetitive movements, or withdrawal. Some children reach the point of self-injurious behavior. Those who have developed language may use it perseveratively at these times.

Cognitive Characteristics

Because autism and PDD are pervasive disorders that affect the child's ability to interact effectively with his or her environment, these children are not able to learn effectively from the social and physical world around them. They often are described as being delayed and/or disordered in most areas of cognitive functioning with occasional discrete and circumscribed areas of great ability. They quite often have uneven development across cognitive areas, with better abilities in visual-spatial reasoning and deficits in auditory-linguistic reasoning. Most children with autism and PDD function overall in the mentally retarded range, with an estimated 70% falling in this range. These children are very difficult to assess on standardized intelligence tests, especially in the first few years of life when they have the greatest difficulty relating to others. Some children with autism and PDD have areas of highly advanced ability, well beyond the average child or their own abilities in other areas. Quite often their exceptional abilities are related to spatial, mathematical, or musical function. Some of the more remarkable abilities that have been observed include being able to do mathematical calculations at a remarkable rate, and being able to give the day of the week that a certain date fell, such as June 26, 1952. Other children have been discovered who are able to play complex musical pieces from memory after having heard them only once.

Some individuals with autism and PDD have higher ability across all areas of cognitive development. The pattern of stronger visual-spatial knowledge than auditory-linguistic comprehension also is typically seen with higher functioning individuals. One of the better known adults who has shared her experience of being autistic is Temple Grandin. She has a doctorate in animal husbandry and is a world-renowned authority on cattle behavior and humane management. Interestingly, she describes her ability to design handling equipment by visualizing the finished product. Then she imagines how it would look and feel from the cow's point of view (Grandin & Scariano, 1986). Most highly educated individuals with autism or PDD have specialized in areas such as science, computers, and mathematics. As adults they still report great discomfort around others and difficulty interpreting social information.

Assessment

Although characteristics of autism and PDD can be identified in some children in the first few months of life, most children are initially referred for evaluation at about the age of 18 to 24 months, often because they are not developing "speech." When asked about the child's earlier development, parents report difficulties with bonding based on a resistance to cuddling, regulatory behaviors, and daily care routines. Other children present with a normal developmental course until 18 to 24 months of age or even later. At that point language begins to disappear and the child withdraws from others. Children with milder levels of autism and PDD may not be identified until 3 to 4 years of age or even considerably later.

Assessing children with autism or PDD requires finding ways to elicit the abilities they have in spite of the difficulties of relating that are the hallmarks of these disorders. Standardized testing is often difficult and must be used only as a starting point in the assessment. The ability to adapt the standardized presentation to the child and to recognize the limitations of the scores as a result of the child's disability are important in providing accurate information on the child's strengths and needs. Information critical in making the diagnosis and developing a treatment plan is gathered from observations of the child across different activities and from parental reports of patterns of behavior seen over time.

In assessing young children suspected of having autism and PDD, there is a danger of overlooking another disorder that leaves a child so unrelated as to look autistic. Children with severe auditory processing disorders that are not part of autism or PDD may appear unrelated just as children with autism and PDD do. Although the difference may not be apparent during the assessment phase, it will be seen in the rapid and dramatic progress they make in relatedness during therapy.

Another group that presents a difficult differential diagnosis from autism and PDD is children with moderate to severe and profound mental retardation. Young children with mental retardation may have self-stimulatory behaviors and show poor responses to social and communicative interactions. The difference is in the variability of functioning levels across all developmental areas. If you use activities at the appropriate developmental level for a child with mental retardation, the barrier of unrelatedness will fall and the child will show an ability for social responsiveness. A low functioning child with autism and PDD, however, will still resist the "intrusion" of the examiner into play and not respond to social games. The amount of effort required to get an interaction going or maintain it is a barometer of the child's existing capacity for social interactions, regardless of the developmental level with respect to cognition, motor, or other linguistic aspects.

As with any developmental disorder, the assessment of children with autism and PDD is best conducted by a multidisciplinary team. The team should include a speech-language pathologist, psychologist, special educator, occupational therapist, developmental pediatrician, and others as appropriate (e.g., physical therapist, psychiatrist, and audiologist). Although the final diagnosis will be made by the psychologist, developmental pediatrician, or psychiatrist, the information from all professionals is needed to complete the diagnostic picture and to develop an appropriate treatment plan. The actual diagnosis of autism and PDD is based on the criteria listed earlier in DSM-IV. Many professionals use a rating scale to quantify the ratings on the various modalities that may be impaired. A rating scale frequently used by psychologists is the *Childhood Autism Rating Scale* (CARS) (Schopler, Reichler, & Renner, 1988). The CARS rates 15 characteristics of children with autism and PDD similar to those in DSM-IIIR and -IV using a Likert scale from 1 to 4 (with 1 = normal responses and 4 = severely abnormal). The totals from the ratings are compared with ratings for children who have been diagnosed as having autism and PDD. This provides a way of quantifying the severity of the disorder.

The speech-language assessment for children with autism and PDD should establish all of the ways the child communicates, as well as the intentions for communication attempts. A child with autism or PDD can have idiosyncratic ways of communicating. The SLP can look behind behaviors for their communicative intent. Some of this information will come from the evaluation, but most will come from a thorough interview of the parents. Ask them how they know when their child wants something, is frustrated, is enjoying him- or herself, is finished, and so on.

Intervention

Since the 1960s treatments that focus on the specific needs of children with autism and PDD for developing social and communicative contacts have shown success in increasing their ability to interact with others and participate in the social world around them. Around the country several programs have been set up specifically for children with autism and PDD. With the move toward inclusion for children with special needs into more mainstream settings, many of the specific programs are exploring ways to provide typical peer models for their students along with the rest of the program (Harris & Handleman, 1994). Most professionals feel that the optimal setting for learning for children with autism and PDD is one with a strong emphasis on structure and routine. These things are critical to the setting because the children cannot provide them easily for themselves. Their difficulty lies in organizing and interpreting what they take in from around themselves. The goal is to organize the environment as much as possible for them.

Keep in mind that children with autism and PDD are more concrete and more absolute in their thinking than typical age peers. Therefore, the best behavior management style includes clear and powerful consequences, both positive and negative, for the child's behavior (Smith, 1993). The structure of any program should provide clear rules and routine with rituals to begin and end each activity, and gradual transitions from one activity to the next.

In programming for individual children, it is important to consult with parents to plan a menu of possible rewards for good behavior. Rewards can include favorite games and pastimes. Include the child's self-stimulatory behaviors and rigid ways of doing things as legitimate reward activities. Clinicians may want to place limits on these activities or behaviors, for example, making loud noises can only be done while alone or can be engaged in for 2 minutes. Think in terms of how any one activity for any child is limited: an upper limit on television or computer game time.

Another possible group of rewards for a child with autism or PDD can be desired kinds of sensory stimulation. Keep these in mind for eliciting requests as well. Check with the child's occupational therapist for suggestions as to what he or she would enjoy. Play on gross motor equipment also provides great opportunities for building the child's tolerance for, and use of, social eye contact and facial expressions. The child can learn to identify these as signaling positive affect in another person.

Echolalia should not be thought of as a behavior to be extinguished. Find out what purposes it serves for the child. In some instances, these purposes may be targeted for replacement by other behaviors or language. In other cases, they may represent the child's attempts at processing, reminiscing over a previous experience, or self-comfort. You may be able to teach some other language to replace some of these purposes. Otherwise, leave the echolalia and move on.

One goal of intervention for children with autism and PDD is teaching the child to accept and allow small changes in routine (e.g., putting the puzzle pieces back in a different order than usual). Look for places to make small changes wherever possible so that the child learns that deviations from routine are not the end of the world. A later goal will be helping the child make changes in play routines. These will be accomplished by providing demonstrations and encouraging the child to try them. The idea of making changes can be taken further by suggesting novel changes for the child to try. All of this work on accepting change takes an enormous amount of time, but is important for expanding the child's world and, consequently, his or her language.

A child with autism or PDD has disordered social interaction ability. Despite this, most of the children do like social contact of some sort. Many love roughhousing with a parent or sibling, others like to be tickled. The children do not dislike all social contact; they just need it to be somewhat predictable and often need to be the initiators. Their need for control and predictability in social contact are part of the same need in other areas of their lives. The normal range of social interactions and responses is very wide, and for a child who cannot read verbal or nonverbal cues, it must seem erratic, unpredictable, and frightening. The task of intervention, then, is to directly teach comprehension of social cues where possible. In addition intervention should also provide, and teach significant others to provide, positive social interactions so that the child learns how rewarding social interactions can be and they become important to seek out.

Another goal for children with autism and PDD is to learn to accept social and appropriate touch. The "high five" is appropriate for almost any age and many children enjoy it. These social interactions can become rewards for getting a work activity done.

Intervention with children with autism and PDD necessarily includes teaching representational play. Without the ability to symbolize, children with autism and PDD do very little pretending on their own. Develop a play scheme taking into account activities with which the children are familiar and interests they have. For example, if the child liked *Beauty and the Beast*, use Mrs. Potts and Chip to share a pretend drink of tea. Add further steps to the scheme if it engages the child successfully. If not, try other schemes to see if they hold the child's interest better. Ultimately, it will be necessary to choose the scheme that works best, (even though the child may prefer *not* to do pretend at all), and stay with that scheme.

Although a game of hiding objects can be fun for a typically developing toddler, for even an older child with autism or PDD, it apparently looks as though something is being taken away so that he or she cannot have it. The game of hiding things has to be taught. Hide-and-seek, the game of hiding **people**, is even more difficult for children with autism and PDD. To their literal and socially unsophisticated minds, the game must not make sense. However, the children will enjoy the slight suspense of discovering the hidden person once they learn how to play. The children's propensity toward maintaining the whole of a learned play scheme will be evident in their looking in the same places in the same order each time they play the game. This is another opportunity to practice change. The language goals can include calling for another, acknowledging being called, asking *where* questions, and so on.

With the youngest children and those with more severe retardation, language should have as much routine as you try to provide in other aspects of the child's life. A direction given should essentially sound the same each time it is given. It is best to use a normal inflection on the utterance along with a soft voice so as not to overwhelm the child's auditory system. Keep in mind that this child is probably a gestalt language learner so that functor words should not be omitted, although the whole utterance should be short. Maintaining the functors keeps the utterance intact as the child will hear it from others, and therefore increases the chances of it being recognized as familiar across speakers and situations.

As the child gets older and recognizes familiar utterances, the objective might become introducing variety in the way a particular request or comment is made and in what is said in a given situation. These changes will help the child expand comprehension ability and provide the opportunity for some flexibility in the language used if cognitive ability allows.

Some children with autism and PDD never develop spoken language, or develop very little, and must rely on augmented systems to communicate. While some individuals need augmentation for communication throughout their lives, many children need it primarily at a young age to help them initiate expressive language. The visual nature of the systems capitalizes on their visual strengths to help them "break the code" of spoken language or somehow provide them with the Rosetta stone for spoken language.

Depending on the cognitive level of the child, printed words may also be used as a form of communication. Some children with autism and PDD have been observed to be hyperlexic: they learn to read at an early age without any formal instruction. They often start by learning letters and numbers, then learning whole sight words. Reading comprehension often lags behind the ability to identify words, but the printed words can be used to aid language comprehension through association with actions and objects. The development of reading skills opens a channel of communication that can be used across settings and throughout the individual's life.

Case Management Issues

Autism and PDD are heartbreaking disorders for families because of the child's difficulty in responding to the normal social interactions that form the basis of family closeness. Often from birth, children with autism and PDD resist the cuddling and comforting that enhance the closeness of parent and child. The parents feel frustrated because it is so difficult to make contact with their child. As the child grows older, his parents begin to understand him as a person and form a relationship with him based on their ability to understand his world. Often children with autism and PDD show no physical anomalies. Parents and professionals alike feel that, if they could only find the key that unlocks the door to the child, then the bright, social being inside would appear. It is this feeling that can make parents and professionals susceptible to fantastic claims and to anecdotal stories of miraculous cures. There are multiple ways of looking at the core issues involved with children with autism and PDD. Each treatment approach proffered is accompanied by a plausible explanation of the core dysfunction in children with autism and PDD and how this intervention corrects the dysfunction.

There are many treatments for children with autism and PDD that cause controversy. Yet there are parents and professionals who believe in improvement with each approach. One factor that makes evaluating the effectiveness of treatments so difficult is inherent in the diagnosis of autism and PDD itself. It is simply a collection of observable characteristics with no implication of causation. What is effective for one type of child with autism or PDD may not be effective for another child. Therapists can look to including in best treatment practices the aspects of any treatment that may work for a particular child. One treatment that has stirred controversy is auditory integration training (AIT, also referred to as Auditory Enhancement Training [AET] or Audio-Psycho-Phonology). See Chapter 4, the section on Case Management Issues. Parents considering its use for their child should be told it is experimental at this point (ASHA, 1994). Another treatment approach generating controversy is the Lovaas method, which employs intensive, one-to-one behavior therapy for 30 to 40 hours per week. Lovaas has published two longitudinal studies that show a 42% cure rate at ages 7 and 11 years in a follow-up of preschool children who participated in a 40-hour per week intervention for 2 years. Eight of the 19 children in the experimental group were indistinguishable from their peers when evaluated at 11 years of age. Only one child in the two control groups showed similar gains (Lovaas, 1987; McEachin, Smith & Lovaas, 1993). The contoversy over the Lovaas method involves the amount of time and financial resources a family must have to follow the treatment regimen. Studies are currently being conducted to attempt to replicate these results.

The overriding issue in case management for children with autism and PDD is to recognize that each child is unique in his or her interpretation of the world and idiosyncratic in his or her responses to it. Children with autism or PDD do not reveal themselves easily in an initial evaluation. Assessment and problem-solving are ongoing and change over time. If you see a strong, consistent reaction to a particular situation, look for the reasons for that reaction. It involves doing a little detective work (what psychologists call single case study design) to determine what the child is communicating with that behavior. Over time, patterns will emerge that will help in designing future interventions and avoiding potential problem situations. If a parent wants to attempt one of the controversial treatment approaches, help them do their research. Is there empirical evidence that the approach is effective for similar children? Does the emphasis of the treatment and its rationale fit the patterns you have observed in their child? If they decide to follow through with treatment, help them find ways to evaluate the effectiveness of the program for their child. If you find something that works for one child, try to keep this empirical approach for the next child and not get caught up in the passion that surrounds some of the treatment approaches promising a cure for all.

Summary

Autism and the other pervasive developmental disorders are lifelong disabilities. With appropriate intervention, bridges of communication can bring the child into the world of those around him and allow him to share himself with others.

REFERENCES

Abikoff, H. (1985). Efficacy of cognitive training intervention in hyperactive children: A critical review. *Clinical Psychological Review, 5*, 479–512.

Abikoff, H. (1991). Cognitive training in ADHD children: Less to it than meets the eye. *Journal of Learning Disabilities, 24*(4), 205–210.

Achenbach, T., & Edelbrock, C. (1983). *Manual for the Child Behavior Checklist and Revised Child Behavior Profile*. Burlington, VT: University of Vermont, Department of Psychiatry.

Ad Hoc Committee on Auditory Integration and Facilitated Communication. (1994). Auditory integration training. *Asha, 36*, 55–58.

Ainsworth, M., Blehar, M., Waters, E., & Wall, S. (1978). *Patterns of attachment: A psychological study of the strange situation*. Hillsdale, NJ: Lawrence Erlbaum.

American Academy of Pediatrics. (1988). Cocaine emergency. *American Academy of Pediatric News, 14* (3).

American Psychiatric Association. (1980). *Diagnostic and statistical manual of mental disorder* (3rd ed.). Washington, DC: Author.

American Psychiatric Association. (1987). *Diagnostic and statistical manual of mental disorders* (3rd ed., rev.). Washington, DC: Author.

American Psychiatric Association. (1994). *Diagnostic and statistical manual of mental disorders* (4th ed., pp. 66–78). Washington, DC: Author.

American Speech-Language-Hearing Association, Ad Hoc Committee on Auditory Integration and Facilitative Communication. (1994). Auditory integration training. *Asha, 36*, 55–58.

Anastopoulos, A. D., DuPaul, G. J., & Barkley, R. A. (1991). Stimulant medication and parent training therapies for attention deficit-hyperactivity disorder. *Journal of Learning Disabilities, 24*(4), 210–218.

Anderson, S. (1992). Motor and sensory characteristics of fragile X. In B. B. Schopmeyer & F. Lowe (Eds.), *The fragile X child* (pp. 59–70). San Diego, CA: Singular Publishing Group.

Atkins, M. S., & Pelham, W. E. (1991). School-based assessment of attention deficit-hyperactivity disorder. *Journal of Learning Disabilities, 24*(4), 197–204.

Autism Society of America. (1991). Information Packet. [Available from ASA, 7910 Woodmont Ave., Suite 650, Bethesda, MD 20814-3015.]

Axelrod, S. (1983). *Behavior modification for the classroom teacher* (2nd ed.). New York: McGraw-Hill.

Baltaxe, C., & Simmons, J. (1990). The differential diagnosis of communication disorders in child and adolescent psychopathology. *Topics in Language Disorders, 10*(4), 17–31.

Barkley, R. A. (1981). Hyperactivity. In E. J. Mash & L. G. Terdal (Eds.), *Behavioral assessment of childhood disorders*. New York: Guilford Press.

Barkley, R. A. (1982). Specific guidelines for defining hyperactivity in children (attention deficit disorder with hyperactivity). In B. Lahey & A. Kazdin (Eds.), *Advances in clinical child psychology, 5*. New York: Plenum.

Barkley, R., & Cunningham, C. E. (1978). Do stimulant drugs improve the academic performance of hyperkinetic children? A review of outcome research. *Clinical Pediatrics, 17*, 85–92.

Barnes, S., Gutfreund, M., Satterly, D., & Wells, G. (1983). Characteristics of adult speech which predict children's language development. *Child Language, 10*, 65–84.

Batshaw, M. L., & Perret, Y. M. (1992). New threats to development: Alcohol, cocaine and AIDS. In *Children with disabilities: A medical primer* (3rd ed.). Baltimore, MD: Paul H. Brookes.

Batshaw, M. L., Perret, Y. M., & Reber, M. (1992). Autism. In M. L. Batshaw & Y. M. Perret (Eds.), *Children with disabilities: A medical primer* (pp. 407–420). Baltimore, MD: Paul H. Brookes.

Batshaw, M. L., Perret, Y. M., & Shapiro, B. K. (1992). Normal and abnormal development: Mental retardation. In *Children with disabilities: A medical primer* (3rd ed., pp. 259–290). Baltimore, MD: Paul H. Brookes.

Bauman, M. (1993). An interview with Margaret Bauman, continued. *Advocate, 25*(1), 17–18.

Beetz, A., Galla, T., & Condon, M. (1992). *Profiles of communicative functioning at the discourse level in various psychiatric populations*. Unpublished manuscript, Inpatient Child Psychiatric Unit, Johns Hopkins Hospital, Baltimore, MD.

Bell, S. M., & Ainsworth, M. (1972). Infant crying and maternal responsiveness. *Child Development, 43,* 1171–1190.

Berliner, L. (1993). Identifying and reporting suspected child abuse and neglect. *Topics in Language Disorders, 13*(4), 15–24.

Bornstein, P., & Quevillon, R. (1976). The effects of a self-instructional package with overactive preschool boys. *Journal of Applied Behavior Analysis, 9,* 179–188.

Brazelton, T. B. (1984). *Neonatal behavior assessment scale* (2nd ed.). Philadelphia: J. B. Lippincott.

Bronheim, S. (1991). An educator's guide to Tourette syndrome. *Journal of Learning Disabilities, 24*(1), 17–22.

Brooks, N. (1988). Behavioral abnormalities in head injured patients. *Scandinavian Journal of Rehabilitation Medicine, 17,* 41–46.

Bruun, R. (1984). Gilles de la Tourette's syndrome: An overview of clinical experience. *Journal of the American Academy of Child Psychiatry, 23*(2), 126–133.

Bruun, R., Cohen, D., & Leckman, J. (1990). *A guide to the diagnosis and treatment of Tourette syndrome* (pp. 5–31). (Available from Tourette Syndrome Association [TSA], 42-40 Bell Boulevard, Bayside, NY 11361.)

Burd, L. (1992). Educational needs of children with Tourette syndrome. In T. Haerle (Ed.), *Children with Tourette syndrome* (pp. 169–207). Rockville, MD: Woodbine House.

Burd, L., Kauffman, D., & Kerbeshian, J. (1992). Tourette syndrome and learning disabilities. *Journal of Learning Disabilities, 25*(9), 598–604.

Burd, L., Kerbeshian, J., Cook, J., Bornhoeff, D. & Fisher, W. (1988). Tourette syndrome in North Dakota. *Neuroscience and Behavioral Reviews, 12,* 223–228.

Burke, A., Crenshaw, D., Green, J., Schlosser, M., & Strocchia-Rivera, L. (1988). Influence of verbal ability on the expression of aggression in physically abused children. *Journal of American Academy of Child Adolescent Psychiatry, 28*(2), 215–218.

Cantwell, D. P. (1977). Hyperkinetic syndrome. In M. Rutter & L. Hersov (Eds.), *Child psychiatry: Modern approaches.* London: Blackwell Scientific.

Cantwell, D. P. (1983). Diagnostic validity of the hyperactive child (attention deficit disorder with hyperactivity) syndrome. *Psychiatric Developments, 3,* 277–300.

Cantwell, D. P., & Baker, L. (1991). Association between attention deficit-hyperactivity disorder and learning disorders. *Journal of Learning Disabilities, 24*(2), 88–95.

Carlson, V., Cicchetti, D., Barnett, D., & Braunwald, K. (1989). Disorganized/disoriented attachment relationships in maltreated infants. *Developmental Psychology, 25*(4), 525–531.

Chasnoff, I., Burns, W., Schnoll, S., & Burns, K. (1985). Cocaine use in pregnancy. *The New England Journal of Medicine, 313*, 666–669.

Chudley, A., & Hagerman, R. (1987). Fragile X syndrome. *Journal of Pediatrics, 110*(6), 821–831.

Cicchetti, D. (1990). The organization and coherence of sociemotional, cognitive, and representational development: Illustrations through a developmental psychopathology perspective on Down syndrome and child maltreatment. In R. Thompson (Ed.), *Nebraska Symposium on Motivation, Volume 36: Socioemotional Development* (pp. 250–366). Lincoln, NE: University of Nebraska Press.

Cohen, S. (1991). Adapting educational programs for students with head injuries. *Journal of Head Trauma Rehabilitation, 6*(1), 56–63.

Cohen, S., & Beckwith, L. (1979). Preterm infant interaction with the caregiver in the first year of life and competence at age two. *Child Development, 50*, 767–776.

Colligan, N. (1989). Recognizing Tourette syndrome in the classroom. *School Nurse*, 1–4.

Comings, B., & Comings, D. (1985). Tourette syndrome: Clinical and psychological aspects of 250 cases. *American Journal of Human Genetics, 37*, 435–450.

Comings, D. (1990). *Tourette syndrome and human behavior*. Duarte, CA: Hope Press.

Comings, D., & Comings, B. (1984). Tourette syndrome and attention deficit disorder with hyperactivity: Are they genetically related? *Journal of American Academy of Child Psychiatry, 23*(2) 138–146.

Comings, D., & Comings, B. (1987). A controlled study of Tourette syndrome: Attention deficit disorder, learning disorders, and school problems. *Journal of Human Genetics, 41*, 701–741.

Cone-Wesson, B., & Wu, P. (1992). Audiologic findings in infants born to cocaine-abusing mothers. In L. M. Rosetti (Ed.), *Developmental problems of drug-exposed infants* (pp. 25–34). San Diego, CA: Singular Publishing Group.

Conners, C. (1980). *Food additives and hyperactive children*. New York: Plenum.

Conners, C. K. (1989a). *Connors' teacher rating scales*. Toronto: Multi-Health Systems.

Conners, C. K. (1989b). *Connors' parent rating scales*. Toronto: Multi-Health Systems.

Conners, S. (1990). *Specific classroom strategies and techniques for students with Tourette syndrome*. (Available from Tourette Syndrome Association [TSA], 42-40 Bell Boulevard, Bayside, NY 11361.)

Cook, D. S., Petersen, R. C., & Moore, D. T. (1990). *Alcohol, tobacco, and other drugs may harm the unborn*. U.S. Department of Health and Human Services, Office for Substance Abuse Prevention. (Available from Rockwall II, 5600 Fishers Lane, Rockville, MD 20857.)

Copeland, A. P. (1981). The relevance of subject variables in cognitive self-instructional programs for impulsive children. *Behavior Therapy, 12*, 520–529.

Coster, W., & Cicchetti, D. (1993). Research on communicative development of maltreated children: Clinical implications. *Topics in Language Disorders, 13*(4), 25–38.

Coster, W., Gersten, M., Beeghly, M., & Cicchetti, D. (1989). Communicative functioning in maltreated toddlers. *Developmental Psychology, 25*(6), 1020–1029.

Courchesne, E. (1989). Neuroanatomical systems involved in infantile autism: The implications of cerebral abnormalities. In G. Dawson (Ed.), *Autism: Nature, diagnosis and treatment* (pp. 119–143). New York: Guilford Press.

Craighead, W. E. (1982). A brief clinical history of cognitive-behavioral therapy with children. *School Psychology Review, 11*, 5–13.

Crites, L. S., Fischer, K. L., McNeish-Stengel, M., & Siegel, C. J. (1992). Working with families of drug-exposed children: Three model programs. In L. M. Rossetti (Ed.), *Developmental problems of drug-exposed infants* (pp. 13–24). San Diego, CA: Singular Publishing Group.

Crittendon, P. (1989). Teaching maltreated children in preschool. *Topics in Early Childhood Special Education, 9*(2), 16–32.

Cullinan, D., Epstein, M. H., & Silver, L. (1977). Modification of impulsive tempo in learning-disabled pupils. *Journal of Abnormal Child Psychiatry, 5*, 437–444.

Culp, R., Watkins, R., Lawrence, H., Letts, D., Kelly, D., & Rice, M. (1991). Maltreated children's language and speech development: Abused, neglected, and abused and neglected. *First Language, 11*, 377–389.

Dawson, G., & Levy, A. (1989). Reciprocal subcortical-cortical influences in autism. In G. Dawson (Ed.), *Autism: Nature, diagnosis and treatment* (pp. 144–173). New York: Guilford Press.

DePompei, R., & Blosser, J. (1987). Strategies for helping head injured children successfully return to school. *Language, Speech, and Hearing Services in Schools, 18*, 292–300.

DePompei, R., & Blosser, J. (1988). *Let's organize today!* [A calendar of daily cognitive-communication activities for the head injured]. Danville, IL: The Interstate Printers and Publishers.

DePompei, R., & Blosser, J. (1989). The head injured student returns to school: Recognizing and treating deficits. *Topics in Language Disorders, 9*(2), 67–77.

DePompei, R., & Zarski, J. (1989). Families, head injury, and cognitive-communicative impairments: Issues for family counseling. *Topics in Language Disorders, 9*(2), 78–89.

Dixon, S. D., & Bejar, R. (1989). Electroencephalographic findings in neonatal associated maternal cocaine and methamphetamine use: Incidence and clinical correlates. *Journal of Pediatrics, 115*, 770–778.

Douglas, V. I., & Peters, K. G. (1979). Toward a clearer definition of the attentional deficit of hyperactive children. In G. A. Hale & M. Lewis (Eds.), *Attention and the development of cognitive skills*. New York: Plenum.

Drabman, R. S., Spitalnik, P., & O'Leary, K. D. (1973). Teaching self-control to disruptive children. *Journal of Abnormal Psychology, 82*, 10–16.

D'Zurilla, T. J., & Goldfried, M. R. (1971). Problem solving and behavior modification. *Journal of Abnormal Psychology, 78*, 107–126.

Eldridge, R., Sweet, R., Shapiro, A., & Arena, F. (1975). Clinical and genetic observations of 21 families with Gilles de la Tourette syndrome. *Neurology, 25*, 379.

Elmer, E. (1977). A follow-up study of traumatized children. *Pediatrics, 59*, 273–279.

Epstein, M. A., Shaywitz, S. E., Shaywitz, B. A., & Woolston, J. L. (1991). The boundaries of attention deficit disorder. *Journal of Learning Disabilities, 24*(2), 78–86.

Favish, J. (1990). *Helpful techniques to aid the student with Tourette syndrome in the completion of written assignments in the classroom and at home*. (Available from Tourette Syndrome Association [TSA], 42-40 Bell Boulevard, Bayside, NY 11361.)

Feeney, J., & Urbanczyk, A. (1992). *Educational programming following acquired brain injury*. Paper presented at the Annual Conference on Cognitive Rehabilitation, Richmond, VA.

Feingold, B. (1975). *Why your child is hyperactive*. New York: Random House.

Finch, A. J., & Spirito, A. (1980). Use of cognitive training to change cognitive processes. *Exceptional Education Quarterly, 1*(1), 31–39.

Forness, S. R., & Kavale, K. (1991). Social skills deficits as primary learning disabilities: A note on problems with the ICLD diagnostic criteria. *Learning Disabilities Research and Practice, 6*, 44–49.

Fox, L., Long, S., & Langlois, A. (1988). Patterns of language comprehension deficit in abused and neglected children. *Journal of Speech and Hearing Disorders, 53*, 239–244.

Freund, L. (1991, Summer/Fall). Clinical research updates on the female with fragile X. *Fragile X Southeast News*, pp. 4–6.

Gadow, K. D. (1986). *Children on medication: Volume 1. Hyperactivity, learning disabilities, and mental retardation*. Boston: Little, Brown.

Gerber, M. M. (1987). Application of cognitive-behavior therapy in behavioral training methods to teaching basic skills to mildly handicapped elementary school students. In M. C. Wang, M. C. Reynolds, & H. J. Walberg (Eds.), *Handbook of special education research and practice: Volume 1. Learner characteristics and adaptive education*. New York: Pergamon.

Glaze, D. G., Frost, J. D., & Jankovic, J. (1983). Sleep in Gilles de la Tourette's syndrome: Clinical and family study of 50 cases. *Annuals of Neurology, 7*, 41.

Golden, G. (1984). Psychologic and neuropsychologic aspects of Tourette's syndrome. *Neurologic Clinics, 2*, 91–102.

Golden, G., & Hood, O. J. (1982). Tics and tremors. *Pediatric Clinics of North America, 29*, 95–103.

Grandin, T., & Scariano, M. (1986). *Emergence: Labelled autistic*. Novato, CA: Arena.

Gresham, F. M., & Elliott, S. N. (1987). The relationship between adaptive behavior and social skills: Issues in definition and assessment. *The Journal of Special Education, 21*(1), 167–181.

Hagen, C. (1986). Language disorders in head trauma. In J. M. Costello & A. L. Holland (Eds.), *Handbook of Speech and Language Disorders*. San Diego, CA: College-Hill Press.

Hagerman, R. (1992). Medical aspects of the fragile X syndrome. In B. B. Schopmeyer & F. Lowe (Eds.), *The fragile X child* (pp. 19–30). San Diego, CA: Singular Publishing Group.

Hagerman, R., Kemper, M., & Hudson, M. (1985). Learning disabilities and attentional problems in boys with fragile X syndrome. *American Journal of the Disabled Child, 139*, 674–678.

Hagin, R., Bececher, R., Pagano, G., & Kreeger, H. (1982). *Effects of Tourette syndrome on learning*. Raven Press.

Hagin, R., & Kugler, J. (1988). School problems associated withTourette's syndrome. In D. J. Cohen, R. D. Brunn, & J. F. Leckman (Eds.), *Tourette's syndrome and tic disorders: Clinical understanding and treatment* (pp. 223–236). New York: John Wiley

Hall, R. (1980). Cognitive behavior modification and information processing skills of exceptional children. *Exceptional Education Quarterly, 1*(1), 9–15.

Harris, S. L., & Handelman, J. S. (Eds.). (1994). Preschool education program for children with autism. Austin, TX: Pro-Ed.

Ho, H. Z., Glahn, T. J., & Ho, J. C. (1988). The fragile X syndrome. *Developmental Medicine and Child Neurology, 30*, 257.

Hoff-Ginsberg, E. (1989). *Effects of social class and interactive setting on maternal speech.* Paper presented at the biennial meeting of the Society for Research in Child Development, Kansas City, MO.

Hogg, C., Callais, M., & Pellegrini, D. (1986). Treatment of a 7-year-old hyperactive boy with educational problems. *Behavioral Psychotherapy, 14*, 145–161.

Holborrow, P., & Berry, P. A. (1986). A multinational, cross-cultural perspective in hyperactivity. *American Journal of Orthopsychiatry, 56*(2), 320–322.

Howard, J., Beckwith, L., Rodning, C., & Kropenske, V. (1989).The development of young children of substance-abusing parents: Insights from seven years of intervention and research. *Zero to Three, 9*(5), 8–12.

Jennett, B., & Teasdale, C. (1981). *Management of head injuries*. Philadelphia, PA: F.A. Davis.

Kanner, L. (1943). Autistic disturbance of affective contact. *Nervous Child, 2*, 217–250.

Kaye, S. (1992). Occupational therapy for children with fragile X syndrome. In B. B. Schopmeyer & F. Lowe (Eds.), *The fragile X child* (pp. 93–138). San Diego, CA: Singular Publishing Group.

Kazdin, A. E. (1975). *Behavior modification in applied settings.* IL: Dorsey Press.

Kemper, L. B., Hagerman, R., & Altshul-Stark, D. (1988). Cognitive profiles of boys with fragile X syndrome. *American Journal of Medical Genetics, 30*, 191–200.

Kemper, S., & Edwards, L. (1986). Children's expression of causality and their construction of narratives. *Topics in Language Disorders, 7*(1), 11–20.

Kendall, P. C., & Braswell, L. (1982). Cognitive-behavioral self-control therapy for children: A components analysis. *Journal of Consulting and Clinical Psychology, 50*, 672–689.

Kendall, P. C., & Cummings, L. (1988). Thought and action in educational interventions: Cognitive-behavioral approaches. In J. C. Witt, S. N. Elliott, & F. M. Gresham (Eds.), *Handbook of behavior therapy in education*. New York: Plenum.

Kendall, P. C., & Finch, A. J., Jr. (1976). A cognitive-behavioral treatment for impulsivity: A case study. *Journal of Consulting and Clinical Psychology, 44*, 852–857.

Kendall, P. C., & Finch, A. J., Jr. (1978). A cognitive-behavioral treatment for impulsivity: A group comparison study. *Journal of Consulting and Clinical Psychology, 47*, 1107–1108.

King, A., & Ollendick, T. (1984). Gilles de la Tourette's disorder: A review. *Journal of Clinical Child Psychology, 13*(1), 2–9.

Kneedler, R. D. (1980). The use of cognitive training to change social behaviors. *Exceptional Education Quarterly, 1*(1), 65–73.

Kneedler, R. D., & Meese, R. L. (1988). Learning-disabled children. In J. C. Witt, S. N. Elliott, & F. M. Gresham (Eds.), *Handbook of special education: Research and practice: Volume 1. Learner characteristics and adaptive education*. New York: Pergamon.

Knutson, J., & Sullivan, P. (1993). Communicative disorders as a risk factor in abuse. *Topics in Language Disorders, 13*(4), 1–14.

Lachiewicz, A. M., & Gullion, D. (1987). Declining IQ's of young males with fragile X syndrome. *American Journal of Mental Retardation, 92*, 272–278.

Lahey, B. B., & Carlson, C. L. (1991). Validity of the diagnostic category of attention deficit disorder without hyperactivity: A review of the literature. *Journal of Learning Disabilities, 24*(2), 110–120.

Lehr, E. (1990). *Psychological management of traumatic brain injuries in children and adolescents*. Gaithersburg, MD: Aspen.

Lesar, S. (1992). Prenatal cocaine exposure: The challenge to education. In L. M. Rosetti (Ed.), *Developmental problems of drug-exposed infants* (pp. 13–24). San Diego, CA: Singular Publishing Group.

Lewis, K. D., Bennett, B., & Schmeder, N. H. (1989). The care of infants menaced by cocaine abuse. *Maternal Child Nursing, 14*(5), 324–329.

Lloyd, J. (1980). Academic instruction and cognitive behavior modification: The need for attack strategy training. *Exceptional Education Quarterly, 1*(1), 53–64.

Loper, A. B. (1980). Metacognitive development: Implications for cognitive training. *Exceptional Education Quarterly, 1*(1), 1–8.

Loper, A. B., & Murphy, D. M. (1985). Cognitive self-regulatory training for underachieving children. In D. Forrest-Pressley, G. E. MacKinnon, & T. G. Walker (Eds.), *Metacognition, cognition and human performance* (Vol. 2, pp. 168–198). New York: Plenum.

Lovaas, I. (1987). Behavioral treatment and normal educational and intellectual functioning in young autistic children. *Journal of Consulting and Clinical Psychology, 55*, 3–9.

Lowe, F. (1992). Speech and language therapy with the fragile X child. In B. B. Schopmeyer & F. Lowe (Eds.), *The fragile X child* (pp. 139–172). San Diego, CA: Singular Publishing Group.

Lubs, H. (1969). A marker X chromosome. *American Journal of Human Genetics, 21*, 231–244.

Luria, A. (1961). *The role of speech in the regulation of normal and abnormal behaviors*. New York: Liveright.

Lynch, M., & Cicchetti, D. (1991). *Patterns of relatedness in maltreated and nonmaltreated children: Connections among multiple representational models.*

MacDonald, C. C. (1992). Perinatal cocaine exposure: Predictor of an endangered generation. In L. M. Rossetti (Ed.), *Developmental problems of drug-exposed infants* (pp. 1–12). San Diego, CA: Singular Publishing Group.

Main, M., & Solomon, J. (1990). Procedures for identifying infants as disorganized/disoriented during the Ainsworth strange situation. In M. Greenberg, D. Cicchett, & M. Cummings (Eds.), *Attachment during the preschool years* (pp. 121–160). Chicago: University of Chicago Press.

Mash, E., Johnston, C., & Kovitz, K. (1983). A comparison of mother-child interactions of physically abused and non-abused children during play and task situations. *Journal of Clinical Child Psychology, 12*(3), 337–346.

Matthews, W. (1988). Attention deficits and learning disabilities in children with Tourette syndrome. *Psychiatric Annals, 18*(7), 217–219.

McCabe, A., & Peterson, C. (Eds.). (1991). *Developing narrative structure.* Hillsdale, NJ: Lawrence Erlbaum.

McCauley, R., & Swisher, L. (1987). Are maltreated children at risk for speech or language impairment? An unanswered question. *Journal of Speech and Hearing Disorders, 52*, 299–303.

McClennen, S. (1992). Cognitive characteristics, assessment, and intervention in fragile X syndrome. In B. B. Schopmeyer & F. Lowe (Eds.), *The fragile X child* (pp. 33–58). San Diego, CA: Singular Publishing Group.

McConkie-Rosell, A. (1991, Summer/Fall). Finding the gene, what does it really mean? *Fragile X Southeast News*, pp. 1–2.

McEachin, J., Smith, T., & Lovaas, I. (1993). Long-term outcome for children with autism who received early intensive behavioral treatment. *American Journal on Mental Retardation, 97*(4), 359–372.

McKinney, J. (1975). Problem solving strategies in reflective and impulsive children. *Journal of Educational Psychology, 67*, 807–820.

McKinney, J., & Haskins, R. (1980). Cognitive training and the development of problem-solving strategies. *Exceptional Education Quarterly, 1*(1), 41–51.

Meichenbaum, D. (1979). *Cognitive behavior modification.* New York: Plenum.

Meichenbaum, D., & Asarnow, J. (1979). Cognitive-behavioral modification and metacognitive development: Implications for the classroom. In P. C. Kendall & S. D. Hollon (Eds.), *Cognitive behavior interventions: Theory, research and procedures.* New York: Academic Press.

Meichenbaum, D., & Goodman, J. (1971). Training impulsive children to talk to themselves: A means of developing self-control. *Journal of Abnormal Psychology, 77*, 115–126.

Mentis, M., & Prutting, C. (1991). Analysis of topics as illustrated in a head injured and a normal adult. *Journal of Speech and Hearing Research, 34*, 583–595.

Meodor, A., & Ollendick, T. H. (1984). Cognitive behavior therapy with children: An evaluation of its efficacy and clinical utility. *Child and Family Behavior Therapy, 6*(3), 25–44.

Messer, S. B. (1976). Reflection-impulsivity: A review. *Psychological Bulletin, 83*, 1026–1052.

Morisset, C., Barnard, K., Greenberg, M., Booth, C., & Spieker, S. (1990). Environmental influences on early language development: The context of social risk. *Development of Psychopathology, 2*, 127–149.

National Head Injury Foundation (NHIF). (1985). *An educator's manual: What educators need to know about students with traumatic brain injury.* Framington, MA: Author.

O'Brien, M. A., & Obrzut, J. E. (1986). Attention deficit disorder with hyperactivity: Review and implications for the classroom. *Journal of Special Education, 20*(3), 281–295.

Office for Substance Abuse Prevention. (1990). Alcohol, tobacco, and other drugs may harm the unborn. (DHHS Publication No. ADM90-1711). Public Health Service. (Available from Rockwall II, 5600 Fishers Lane, Rockville, MD.)

Palkes, H., Stewart, M. S., & Freedman, J. (1972). Improvement in maze performance of hyperactive boys as a function of verbal-training procedures. *The Journal of Special Education, 5*, 337–342.

Pate, S. (1993). *Language assessment and intervention*. Presentation at the annual convention of the Council for Learning Disabilities, Baltimore, MD.

Powers, M. D. (Ed.). (1989). *Children with autism: A parents' guide*. Rockville, MD: Woodbine House.

Prigatano, G., & Klonoff, D. (1988). Psychotherapy and neuropsychological assessment after brain injury. *Journal of Head Trauma Rehabilitation, 3*, 45–56.

Prizant, B. (1992). *Socioemotional considerations in assessment and intervention*. Paper presented at Conference for Learning Disabilities, Baltimore, MD.

Prizant, B., & Wetherby, A. (1989). Enhancing language and communication in autism: From theory to practice. In G. Dawson (Ed.), *Autism: Nature, diagnosis and treatment* (pp. 282–309). New York: Plenum.

Prouty, L. A., Rogers, C., & Stevenson, R. E. (1988). Fragile X syndrome: Growth, development and intellectual function. *American Journal of Medical Genetics, 30*, 123.

Randall, T. (1992). Infants, children test positive for cocaine after exposure to second-hand crack smoke. *Journal of the American Medical Association, 267*(8), 1044–1045.

Reiss, A. L., & Freund L. (1990). Fragile X syndrome. *Biological Psychiatry, 27*, 223.

Rivers, M., & Hedrick, D. (1992). Language and behavioral concerns for drug-exposed infants and todddlers. In L. M. Rossetti (Ed.), *Developmental problems of drug-exposed infants* (pp. 63–73). San Diego, CA: Singular Publishing Group.

Roddy, S. (1989). Bad habit, simple tic, or Tourette syndrome? *Contemporary Pediatrics, 6*, 22–35.

Rosenberg, M. (1985). Advances in educating students with special educational needs: A view from the United States. *Westminster Studies in Education, 8*, 77–96.

Rosenberg, M. S., Sindeler, P. T., & Stedt, J. (1985). The effects of supplemented on-task contingencies upon the acquisition of simple and difficult academic test. *Journal of Special Education, 19*, 189–203.

Rosenthal, M., & Muir, C. (1983). Methods of family intervention. In M. Rosenthal, E. R. Griffith, M. R. Bond, & J. D. Miller (Eds.), *Rehabilitation of the head injured adult* (pp. 407–418). Philadelphia, PA: F. A. Davis.

Rossetti, L. M. (1992). *Developmental problems of drug-exposed infants*. San Diego, CA: Singular Publishing Group.

Rousseau, F., Heitz, D., & Biancalana, V. (1991). Direct diagnosis by DNA analysis of the fragile X syndrome of mental retardation. *New England Journal of Medicine, 325*, 1673.

Routh, D. K. (1980). Developmental aspects of hyperactivity. In C. K. Whalen & B. Henker (Eds.), *Hyperactive children: The social ecology of identification and treatment*. New York: Academic Press.

Russell, N. (1993). Educational considerations in traumatic brain injury: The role of the speech-language pathologist. *Language, Speech, and Hearing Services in Schools, 24*(2), 67–76.

Sameroff, A., & Fiese, B. (1990). Transitional regulation and early intervention. In S. Meisels & J. Shonkoff (Eds.), *Early intervention: A handbook of theory, practice and analysis*. New York: Cambridge University Press.

Santostefano, S. (1978). *A biodevelopmental approach to clinical child psychology*. New York: John Wiley.

Savage, R. (1991). Identification, classification, and placement issues for students with traumatic brain injuries. *Journal of Head Trauma Rehabilitation, 6*(1), 1–9.

Scharfenaker, S. K. (1990). The fragile X syndrome. *Asha, 31*(9) 45–47.

Schloss, P. J., Schloss, C. N., Wood, C. E., & Kiehl, W. S. (1990). A critical review of social skills research with behaviorally disordered students. *Behavioral Disorders, 12*, 11–15.

Schopler, E., Reicher, R., & Renner, B. (1988). *The Childhood Autism Rating Scale* (CARS). Los Angeles: Western Psychology Services.

Singer, H., & Walkup, J. (1991). Tourette syndrome and other tic disorders: Diagnosis, pathophysiology, and treatment. *Medicine, 70*(1), 15–31.

Smith, T. (1993). Autism. In T. R. Giles (Ed.), *Handbook of effective psychotherapy* (pp. 107–131). New York: Guilford Press.

Snow, C. (1977). The development of conversation between mothers and babies. *Journal of Child Language, 4*, 1–22.

Snow, C., Midkiff-Borundo, S., Small, A. & Proctor, A. (1984). Therapy as social interaction: Analyzing the contexts for language remediation. *Topics in Language Disorders, 4*(4), 72–85.

Sohlberg, M., & Mateer, C. (1989). A process specific approach to cognitive rehabilitation. In M. Sohlberg & C. Mateer (Eds.), *Introduction to cognitive rehabilitation*. New York: Guilford Press.

Sparks, S. N. (1993). *Children of prenatal substance abuse*. San Diego, CA: Singular Publishing Group.

Steff, M. (1984). Mental health needs associated with Tourette's syndrome. *American Journal of Public Health, 74*, 1310–1313.

Streissguth, A., Aase, J., Clarren, S., Randels, S., LaDue, R., & Smith, D. (1991). Fetal alcohol syndrome in adolescents and adults. *Journal of the American Medical Association, 265,* 1961–1967.

Sutherland, G. R., & Mulley, S. C. (1990). Diagnostic molecular genetics of the fragile X. *Clinical Genetics, 37,* 2.

Szatmari, P., Offord, D. R., & Boyle, M. H. (1989). Ontario child health study: Prevalence of attention deficit disorder with hyperactivity. *Journal of Child Psychology and Psychiatry, 30*(2), 219–230.

Teasdale, G., & Jennett, B. (1974). Assessment of coma and impaired consciousness: A practical scale. *Lancet, 2,* 81–83.

Torup, E. (1972). A follow-up study of children with tics. *Acta Paediatrica Scandinavica, 51,* 261–268.

Trace, R. (1992). Recognize and report child abuse. *Advance,* 7–11.

U.S. General Accounting Office Report to the Chairman, Committee on Finance, U.S. Senate. (1990). *Drug exposed infants: A generation at risk* (GAO/HRD Publication No. 90-138). Washington, DC: Government Printing Office.

Volkmar, F. (1989). Medical problems, treatments, and professionals. In M. Powers (Ed.), *Children with autism: A parents' guide* (pp. 55–78). Rockville, MD: Woodbine House.

Vygotsky, L. (1962). *Thought and language.* New York: John Wiley.

Waaland, P., & Cockrell, J. (1990). *Pediatric traumatic brain injury* (Special Topic Report No. 3), Richmond, VA: Rehabilitation Research & Training Center on Severe Traumatic Brain Injury.

Warren, B. (1992, November). *The importance of speech pathology in psychiatry.* Paper presented at the annual convention of the American Speech-Language-Hearing Association, San Antonio, TX.

Whalen, C. K., & Henker, B. (1987). Cognitive behavior therapy for hyperactive children: What do we know? *Journal of Children in Contemporary Society, 19*(2), 123–141.

Whalen, C. K., & Henker, B. (1991). Social impact of stimulant treatment for hyperactive children. *Journal of Learning Disabilities, 24*(4), 231–241.

Whalen, C., Henker, B., & Hinshaw, S. (1985). Cognitive behavior therapies for hyperactive children: Premises, problems, and prospects. *Journal of Abnormal Psychology, 13*(3), 391–410

Williams, J., & Ellsworth, N. (1990). Teaching learning disabled adolescents to think critically using a problem-solving schema. *Exceptionality, 1,* 135–146.

Wolfe, D. (1987). *Child abuse.* Newbury Park, CA: Sage.

Wong, B. Y. L. (1985b). Issues in cognitive-behavioral interventions in academic skill areas. *Journal of Abnormal Child Psychology, 13*, 425–441.

Ylvisaker, M., Szekeres, S., Henry, K., Sullivan, D., & Wheeler, P. (1987). Topics in cognitive rehabilitation therapy. In M. Ylvisaker & E. M. Gobble (Eds.), *Community re-entry for head injured adults*. Boston, MA: College-Hill Press.

APPENDIX A

Resources for Traumatic Brain Injury

Organizations

Alabama

Alabama Head Injury Foundation
P.O. Box 550008
Birmingham, AL 35255
(205) 328-3505
(800) 433-8002 (in state)

Arizona

Arizona Head Injury Foundation
630 N. Craycroft Road, Suite 139
Tucson, AZ 85711-1441
(602) 747-7140
(800) 432-3465 (in state)

Arkansas

Arkansas Head Injury Foundation
P.O. Box 7138
Sherwood, AR 72116
(800) 235-2443

California

California Head Injury Foundation
8060 Florence Avenue, Suite 302
Downey, CA 90240
(310) 803-4418

Colorado

Colorado Head Injury Foundation
5601 S. Broadway, Suite 350
Littleton, CO 80121
(303) 730-7112
(800) 955-2443 (in state)

Connecticut

Connecticut Traumatic Brain Injury Association
1800 Silas Deane Highway, Suite 224
Rocky Hill, CT 06067
(203) 721-8111
(800) 278-8242 (in state)

Delaware

Delaware Head Injury Foundation
P.O. Box 9876
Newark, DE 19714
(302) 654-7705

Florida

Florida Head Injury Association
North Broward Medical Center
201 E. Sample Road
Pompano Beach, FL 33064
(305) 786-2400
(800) 992-3442 (in state)

Georgia

Georgia Head Injury Association
1441 Clifton Road #215
Atlanta, GA 30322
(404) 727-5588

Illinois

Illinois Head Injury Association
8903 Burlington Avenue
Brookfield, IL 60513
(708) 485-2080
(800) 284-4442 (in state)

Indiana

Head Injury Foundation/Indiana
East 16th Street, Suite B5
Indianapolis, IN 46218
(317) 356-7722
(800) 407-4246 (Helpline)

Iowa

Iowa Head Injury Association
2101 Kimball Avenue, LL7
Waterloo, IA 50702
(319) 291-3552
(800) 475-4442 (in state)

Kansas

Head Injury Association of Kansas and Greater Kansas City
1100 Pennsylvania, Suite 305
Kansas City, MO 64105-1336
(816) 842-8607
(800) 783-1356

Kentucky

Kentucky Head Injury Association
3910 Dupont Square South, Suite D
Louisville, KY 40207-4648
(502) 899-7141

Louisiana

Louisiana Head Injury Foundation
1001 Howard Avenue, Suite 2101
New Orleans, LA 70113
(504) 558-0051

Maine

Maine Head Injury Foundation
P.O. Box 2224
Augusta, ME 04338-2224
(207) 626-0022

Maryland

Maryland Head Injury Foundation
916 S. Rolling Road
Baltimore, MD 21228
(410) 747-7758
(800) 221-NHIF (in state)

Massachusetts

Massachusetts Head Injury Association
Denholm Building
484 Main Street
Worcester, MA 01608
(508) 795-0244
(800) 242-0030 (in state)

Michigan

Michigan Head Injury Alliance
8137 W. Grand River, Suite A
Brighton, MI 48116
(810) 229-5880
(800) 772-4323 (in state)

Minnesota

Minnesota Head Injury Association
12 Colonial Office Park
2700 University Avenue West
St. Paul, MN 55114
(612) 644-1121
(800) 669-MHIA (in state)

Mississippi

Mississippi Head Injury Association
P.O. Box 55912
Jackson, MS 39296-5912
(601) 981-1021

Missouri

Missouri Head Injury Association
P.O. Box 84
Jefferson City, MO 65109
(314) 893-2444

Montana

Montana Head Injury Association
Institute for Health and Human Services
Eastern Montana College
1500 N. 30th Street, Room 235
Billings, MT 59101-0298
(406) 657-2077

Nebraska

Nebraska Head Injury Association
P.O. Box 397
Route 1, Box 132
Milford, NE 68405
(402) 761-2781
(800) 743-4781 (in state)

New Hampshire

NHIF/New Hampshire Association
2½ Beacon Street, Suite 171
Concord, NH 03301
(603) 225-8400

New Jersey

New Jersey Head Injury Association
1090 King George Post Road #708
Edison, NJ 08837-3722
(908) 738-1002

New Mexico

New Mexico Head Injury Foundation
2819 Richmond, N.E.
Albuquerque, NM 87107
(505) 889-8008
(800) 279-7480 (in state)

New York

New York State Head Injury Association
855 Central Avenue
Albany, NY 12206-1506
(518) 459-7911
(800) 228-8201 (in state)

North Carolina

North Carolina Head Injury Foundation
301 South Tryon Street, Suite 1710
Charlotte, NC 28282
(704) 332-9834
(800) 377-1464 (in state)

North Dakota

Head Injury Association of North Dakota
2111 E. Main Avenue, Suite 14
West Fargo, ND 58708
(701) 281-0527
(800) 279-6344 (in state)

Ohio

The Ohio Head Injury Association
1335 Dublin Road, Suite 50A
Columbus, OH 43215-1000
(614) 481-7100
(800) 686-9563 (in state)

Oklahoma

Oklahoma Head Injury Foundation
P.O. Box 3225
Tulsa, OK 74101-3225
(405) 556-0147

Oregon

Oregon Head Injury Foundation
P.O. Box 40275
Eugene, OR 97404
(503) 689-7310

South Carolina

South Carolina Head Injury Association
P.O. Box 1912
Orangeburg, SC 29116
(803) 533-1613
(800) 767-9701 (in state)

Tennessee

Tennessee Head Injury Association
P.O. Box 1090
Hendersonville, TN 37077-1090
(615) 264-3052

Texas

Texas Head Injury Association
Plaza 290 Office Building, Suite 301
6633 East Highway 290
Austin, TX 78723
(512) 467-6872
(800) 392-0040 (in state)

Utah

Utah Head Injury Association
1800 S. West Temple, Suite 208
Salt Lake City, UT 84115
(801) 484-2240
(800) 281-8442 (in state)

Vermont

Vermont Association/NHIF
P.O. Box 1837, Station A
Rutland, VT 05701
(802) 446-3017

Virginia

Virginia Head Injury Foundation
3212 Cutshaw Avenue, Suite 315
Richmond, VA 23230
(804) 355-5748
(800) 334-8443 (in state)

Washington

Washington State Head Injury Foundation
300 120th Avenue, N.E.
Building 3, Room 131
Bellevue, WA 98005
(206) 451-0000
(800) 523-LIFT (in state)

West Virginia

West Virginia Head Injury Foundation
P.O. Box 574
Institute, WV 25112-0574
(304) 766-4892
(800) 356-6443

Wisconsin

Wisconsin Brain Trauma Association
735 N. Water Street, Suite 701
Milwaukee, WI 53202
(414) 271-7463

Wyoming

Wyoming Head Injury Association
246 South Center, Suite 206
Casper, WY 82601
(307) 473-1767
(800) 643-6457 (Nationwide)

Materials for Parents and Professionals

Blosser, J., & DePompei, R. (1994). *Pediatric traumatic brain injury*. San Diego, CA: Singular Publishing Group.

Deaton, A. (1987). *Pediatric head trauma guide for families.* (Available from Cumberland Hospital, P.O. Box 150, New Kent, VA 23124.)

Lash, M. (1991). *When your child is seriously injured: The emotional impact on families*. NJ: Exceptional Parent.

Lash, M. (1992). *When your child goes to school after an injury*. NJ: Exceptional Parent.

Mira, M., Tucker, B., & Tyler, J. (1992). *Traumatic head injury in children and adolescents: A sourcebook for teachers and other school personnel.* Austin, TX: Pro-Ed.

Palfrey, J. (1992). *Working toward a balance in our lives: A booklet for families of children with disabilities and special health care needs*. Boston, MA: Project School Care.

Raines, S., & Waaland, P. (1991). *For kids only: A guide to brain injury.* Richmond, VA: RRTC Medical College of Virginia.

Savage, R., & Wolcott G. (1994). *Educational Dimensions of Acquired Brain Injury*. Austin, TX: Pro-Ed.

Williams, J., & Kay, T. (1991). *Head Injury: A family matter*. Baltimore, MD: Paul H. Brookes.

APPENDIX B

Resources for Attention Deficit Disorder

Organizations

Alabama

Ch.A.D.D. of Birmingham
Birmingham, AL
(205) 871-1100

Ch.A.D.D. of Central Alabama
Montgomery, AL
(205) 281-1871

Ch.A.D.D. of Gadsden-Etowah
Gadsden, AL
(205) 492-9399

Ch.A.D.D. of Mobile
Mobile, AL
(205) 633-3229

Arizona

Arizona Association for Learning Disabilities
815 E. Camelback Road, Suite 108
Phoenix, AZ 85014
(602) 949-7112

Arizona Council on Behalf of Children and Adults with Attention Deficit Disorders
3881 West Sunny Shadows
Tucson, AZ 85741

Ch.A.D.D. of Bullhead City
Bullhead City, AZ
(602) 758-8628

Ch.A.D.D. of Flagstaff
Flagstaff, AZ
(602) 744-6364

West Valley ADD
Glendale Library
59th and Brown
Glendale, AZ 85502
(602) 492-0919

Arkansas

Learning Disabilities Association of Arkansas
P.O. Box 7316
Little Rock, AR 72216
(501) 666-8777

California

California Association for Children and Adults with Learning Disabilities
17 Buena Vista Avenue
Mill Valley, CA 94941
(415) 383-5242

North County Parents Organization for Children with Special Needs
3088 East Live Oak Park Road
Fallbrook, CA 92028-2611
(619) 723-8787 (help line)

Ch.A.D.D. of Chula Vista
Chula Vista, CA
(619) 585-4614

Ch.A.D.D. of San Diego
San Diego, CA
(619) 569-9546

Ch.A.D.D. of Sonoma County
Penngrove, CA
(707) 664-1521

Colorado

Colorado Association for Children and Adults with Learning Disabilities
P.O. Box 32188
Aurora, CO 80041

ADDAG of Berthoud
Berthoud, CO
(303) 532-4071

ADDAG of Brighton
Brighton, Co.
(303) 659-5790

ADDAG of Greeley
Greeley, CO
(303) 351-7314

Connecticut

Ch.A.D.D. of Greater Hartford/New Britain
682 Prospect Avenue
Hartford, CT 06105
(203) 236-1343

Connecticut Association for Children and Adults with Learning Disabilities
18 Marshall Street
South Norwalk, CT 06854
(203) 838-5010

Delaware

Newcastle County Association for Children and Adults with Learning Disabilities
P.O. Box 577
Bear, DE 19701
(302) 994-0707

District of Columbia

District of Columbia Association for Children and Adults with Learning Disabilities
P.O. Box 6350
Washington, DC 20015
(202) 244-5177

Florida

ADD-UP
392 Glenbrook Drive
Lantana, FL 33462
(407) 968-7126

Ch.A.D.D. of Brevard County
900 Mandarin Drive, N.E.
Palm Bay, FL 32905
(407) 676-2804

Georgia

Ch.A.D.D. of Cobb County
Roswell, GA
(404) 992-7067

Ch.A.D.D. of Decatur
Decatur, GA
(404) 458-5651

Ch.A.D.D. of Gainesville
Gainesville, GA
(404) 536-6898

Ch.A.D.D. of North Atlanta
Atlanta, GA
(404) 921-6155

Hawaii

Hawaii Association forChildren and Adults with Learning Disabilities
Room 103, 200 North Vineyard
Honolulu, HI 96817
(808) 536-9684

Idaho

A.D.D. Support Group
8420 Holbrook Court
Boise, ID 83704
(208) 327-0624

Illinois

Illinois Association for Children and Adults with Learning Disabilities
20 East Jackson, Room 900
Chicago, IL 60604
(312) 663-9535

Illinois Association for Hyperactivity and ADD
507 Thornhill Drive
Carol Stream, IL 60188
(312) 653-0222

Ch.A.D.D. of Chicago North
Chicago, IL
(312) 525-5233

Ch.A.D.D. of Peoria
Peoria, IL
(309) 674-8388

Indiana

Guidance for Living with ADD (GLADD)
P.O. Box 55613
Indianapolis, IN 46205
(317) 259-1827
(317) 257-6160

Ch.A.D.D. of Southern Indiana
Evansville, IN
(812) 867-7056

Iowa

Attention Deficit Disorder—Understanding Parents (ADD-UP)
3034 Sweetbriar
Iowa City, IA 52245
(319) 351-2520

Support Group for Parents of Children with ADD
5114 Gordon Avenue, N.W.
Cedar Rapids, IA 52405
(319) 396-5239

Kansas

Kansas Association for Adults and Children with Learning Disabilities
P.O. Box 4424
Topeka, KS 66604
(913) 234-9336

Kentucky

ADD Parent Support Group
c/o Our Lady of Peace Hospital
2020 Newbury Road
Louisville, KY 40232
(502) 896-2612

Kentucky Association for
Children and Adults with
Learning Disabilities
2233 Alta Avenue
Louisville, KY 40205
(502) 451-8011

Louisiana

Ch.A.D.D. of Acadiana
Lafayette, LA
(318) 984-7167
Ch.A.D.D. of St. Tammany Parish
Mandeville, LA
(504) 626-5166

Ch.A.D.D. of Southwest Louisiana
Sulphur, LA
(318) 625-8805

Maine

Special Needs Parent Information Network (SPIN)
P.O. Box 2967
Augusta, ME 04330
(800) 325-0220

Maryland

Attention Deficit Disorder Support Group of Howard County, Maryland
9222 Mellenbrook Road
Columbia, MD 21045
(410) 992-7550

Ch.A.D.D. of Baltimore County
28 Allegheny Avenue, Suite 1208
Towson, MD 21204
(410) 828-5300

Metropolitan Baltimore Association for Children and Adults with Learning Disabilities
320 Maryland National Bank Building
Baltimore, MD 21202
(410) 252-9053

Ch.A.D.D. of Southern Maryland
Mechanicsville, MD
(301) 373-3609

Ch.A.D.D. of Towson
Baltimore, MD
(410) 665-0990

Massachusetts

ADD Parent Support Group Network
47 Kristin Road
Plymouth, MA 02360
(508) 746-3959
(508) 746-7093

New England Attention Disorder (NEAD)
P.O. Box 82
Northboro, MA 01532
(508) 393-8039

Ch.A.D.D. of Northern Massachusetts
Dracut, MA
(508) 957-0653

Ch.A.D.D. of Western Massachusetts
Greenfield, MA
(413) 586-1877

Michigan

ADD Association of Michigan
P.O. Box 9037
Livonia, MI 48154
(313) 464-8233

Michigan Association for Children and Adults with Learning Disabilities
20777 Randall
Farmington, MI 48024
(313) 471-0790

Ch.A.D.D. of Central Michigan
Big Rapids, MI
(616) 796-0090

Ch.A.D.D. of Southwest Michigan
Schoolcraft, MI
(616) 679-4174

Minnesota

Minnesota Association for Children and Adults with Learning Disabilities
#494-N
1821 University Avenue
St. Paul, MN 55104
(612) 646-6136

Mississippi

Mississippi Association for Children and Adults with Learning Disabilities
P.O. Box 9387
Jackson, MS 39206
(601) 982-2812

Ch.A.D.D. of Central Mississippi
Pearl, MS
(601) 932-1598

Ch.A.D.D. of Mississippi Gulf Coast
Gulfport, MS
(601) 832-8347

Missouri

Missouri Association for Children and Adults with Learning Disabilities
P.O. Box 3303
2740 South Glenstone
Springfield, MO 65808
(417) 864-5110

Gateway Ch.A.D.D.
Maryland Heights, MO
(314) 298-1621

Ch.A.D.D. of Mid Missouri
Columbia, MO
(314) 445-7273

Ch.A.D.D. of the State Fair Area
Sedalia, MO
(816) 827-3540

Montana

Montana Association for Children and Adults with Learning Disabilities
3024 Macona Lane
Billings, MT 59102
(406) 252-4845

Parents Let's Unite for Kids (P.L.U.K.)
EMC MCHC
1500 North 30th
Billings, MT 59101
(406) 657-2055

Nebraska

Nebraska Association for Children and Adults with Learning Disabilities
P.O. Box 6464
Omaha, NE 68106
(402) 571-7771

Nevada

Nevada Association for the Handicapped
6200 West Oakley
Las Vegas, NV 89102
(702) 870-7050

New Hampshire

New Hampshire Association for Children and Adults with Learning Disabilities
20 Wedgewood Drive
Concord, NH 03307
(603) 224-5872

Ch.A.D.D. of Central New Hampshire
Dunbarton, NH
(603) 224-4153

New Jersey

Atlantic County Association for Children and Adults with Learning Disabilities
P.O. Box 3241
Margate, NJ 08402
(609) 822-4082

Ch.A.D.D. of Central New Jersey
Belle Mead, NJ
(908) 874-3124

Ch.A.D.D. of South Jersey
Cherry Hill, NJ
(609) 482-1654

New Mexico

ADD Support Group
c/o Mountain Elementary School
2280 North Road
Los Alamos, NM 87544-1798
(505) 662-4367

New York

New York Association for the Learning Disabled
155 Washington Avenue
Albany, NY 12210
(518) 436-4633

Ch.A.D.D. of Central New York
Syracuse, NY
(315) 476-6489

Ch.A.D.D. of New York City
Manhattan, NY
(212) 724-9499

Ch.A.D.D. of Queens County
Queens, NY
(718) 272-0627

Ch.A.D.D. of Westchester County
White Plains, NY
(914) 763-5094

North Carolina

Learning Disabilities Association of North Carolina
P.O. Box 3542
Chapel Hill, NC 27515-3542
(919) 967-9537

Ch.A.D.D. of Coastal Carolina
Wilmington, NC
(919) 791-8834

Ch.A.D.D. of Western North Carolina
Asheville, NC
(704) 274-7562

North Dakota

North Dakota Learning Disabilities Association
7 E. Central Avenue, #202
Minot, ND 58701
(701) 852-5525

Ohio

Ohio Association for Children and Adults with Learning Disabilities
2800 Euclid Avenue #25
Cleveland, OH 44115
(216) 861-6665

Ch.A.D.D. of Central Ohio
Worthington, OH
(614) 888-3241

Ch.A.D.D. of Richland County
Mansfield, OH
(419) 589-5511, Ext. 286

Oklahoma

Oklahoma Association for Children and Adults with Learning Disabilities
3701 Northwest 62nd
Oklahoma City, OK 73112
(405) 943-9434

Oregon

Oregon Association for Children and Adults with Learning Disabilities
Portland State University
PSU Box 751
Portland, OR 97207
(503) 229-4439

Pennsylvania

Ch.A.D.D. of Bucks County
14 Putnam Drive
Holland, PA 18966
(215) 968-3430

Ch.A.D.D. of Lancaster County
Lancaster, PA
(717) 569-3387

Ch.A.D.D. of the Capitol Area
Carlisle, PA
(717) 243-9576

Rhode Island

Rhode Island Association for Children and Adults with Learning Disabilities
P.O. Box 6685
Providence, RI 02904

South Carolina

Piedmont Association for Children and Adults with Learning Disabilities
P.O. Box 262
Greenwood, SC 29648
(803) 229-7229

South Dakota

Ch.A.D.D. of South Dakota
P.O. Box 84813
Sioux Falls, SD 57118
(605) 335-8844

Tennessee

Ch.A.D.D. of Greater Memphis
Memphis, TN
(901) 795-0111

Tennessee Association for Children and Adults with Learning Disabilities
P.O. Box 281028
Memphis, TN 38128
(901) 323-1430

Texas

Attention Deficit Hyperactivity Disorder (ADHD) Association of Texas
P.O. Box 61592
Houston, TX 77208-1592
(713) 955-3720

Texas Association for Children and Adults with Learning Disabilities
1011 West 31st Street
Austin, TX 78705
(512) 458-8234

Ch.A.D.D. of Texarkana
Texarkana, TX
(214) 792-9600

Utah

It All Adds Up!/Attention Deficit Disorder Foundation
P.O. Box 1082
Sandy, UT 84091-1082
(801) 571-5463

Vermont

Vermont Association for the Learning Disabled
Nine Heaton Street
Montpelier, VT 05602
(802) 223-5480

Ch.A.D.D. of Upper Valley
Norwich, VT
(802) 649-2424

Virginia

Parent/Teacher Support Group—Hyperactive Attention Deficit (HADD)
106 South Street, #207
Charlottesville, VA 22901
(804) 979-5771

Washington

Washington Association for Children and Adults with Learning Disabilities
17530 Northeast Union Hill Road, Suite 100
Redmond, WA 98052
(206) 882-0792

West Virginia

Ch.A.D.D. of Eastern Panhandle
Harpers Ferry, WV
(304) 725-6473

Wisconsin

Wisconsin Association for Hyperactive Children
P.O. Box 1477
Milwaukee, WI 53201-1477
(414) 332-6172

Wyoming

ADDAG of Wyoming
(307) 721-4742

Materials for Parents and Professionals

Friedman, R., & Doyal, G. (1987). *Attention deficit disorder and hyperactivity*. Danville, IL: The Interstate Printers and Publishers.

Goldstein, D.,& Goldstein, M. (1989). *A parent's guide: Attention deficit-hyperactivity disorder in children*. Salt Lake City, UT: Neurology, Learning and Behavior Center.

Hart, L. (1989). *The winning family*. Oakland, CA: Life Skills Press.

Lifson, A. (1980). *Taming the tornado*. Costa Mesa, CA: Educational Consultant Group Publications.

Turecki, S., & Tonner, L. (1985). *The difficult child*. New York: Bantam Books.

Wender, P. (1987). *The hyperactive child, adolescent and adult: Attention deficit disorder through the life span*. New York: Oxford University Press.

Cima, C. *Coping with the hyperactive child*. (Available from Learning Disabilities Association, 4156 Library Rd., Pittsburgh, PA 15234.)

Ente, G. *Guidelines for living with a hyperactive child*. (Available from Learning Disabilities Association, 4156 Library Rd., Pittsburgh, PA 15234.)

Silver, L. B. *Attention deficit disorders* (for parents). (Available from Learning Disabilities Association, 4156 Library Rd., Pittsburgh, PA 15234.)

Silver, L. B. *Attention deficit disorders* (for teachers). (Available from Learning Disabilities Association, 4156 Library Rd., Pittsburgh, PA 15234.)

Coleman, W. S. *Attention deficit disorders and hyperactivity*. (Available from Learning Disabilities Association, 4156 Library Rd., Pittsburgh, PA 15234.)

Goldstein, S. (1989). *Why won't my child pay attention?* [Video]. (Available from Neurology, Learning and Behavior Center, 230 South 500 East, Suite 100, Salt Lake City, UT 84102.)

APPENDIX C

Resources for Tourette Syndrome

Organizations

Alabama

TSA-Alabama Chapter
(serves entire state)
For current phone number,
contact national TSA.

Alabama Association for
Children and Adults with
Learning Disabilities (ACLD)
P.O. Box 11588
Montgomery, AL 36111
(205) 277-9151

Alaska

Alaska Tourette Syndrome Association
9440 Chenega Dr.
Anchorage, AK 99507
(907) 333-0969
(907) 337-1583

Arizona

Arizona Tourette Syndrome Association
342 W.Shaw Butte Drive
Phoenix, AZ 85029
(602) 993-1573

Arkansas

TSA-Arkansas Chapter
(serves entire state)
For current phone number, contact national TSA.

Association for Children and Adults with Learning Disabilities (ACLD)
P.O. Box 705
Hope, AR 71801
(501) 777-5572

Association for Child and Adults with Learning Disabilities
State Office
P.O. Box 7316
Little Rock, AR 72217
(501) 666-8777

California

TSA-Northern California Chapter
(serves Eureka, Fresno, Marysville, North Redding, Bay, Oakland, Sacramento, Salinas, San Francisco, San Jose, and Stockton)
For current phone number, contact national TSA.

TSA-Southern California Chapter
(serves Alhambra, Bakersfield, Englewood, Long Beach, Los Angeles, Oxnard, Pasadena, Santa Ana, San Bernardino, San Diego, Van Nys, and Wojave)
For current phone number, contact national TSA.

Tourette Syndrome Clinic
Department of Medical Genetics
City of Hope National Medical Center
Duarte, CA 91010
(818) 359-8111, ext.2631
(818) 357-7624

Association for Children and Adults with Learning Disabilities (ACLD)
State Office
17 Buena Vista Ave.
Mill Valley, CA 94941
(415) 383-5242

Colorado

TSA-Colorado Chapter
(serves entire state)
For current phone number,
contact national TSA.

Colorado Association for Children with Learning Disabilities (ACLD)
1835 Cherry
Denver, CO 80220
(303) 973-3134
State Office ACLD
P.O.Box 32188
Aurora, CO 80041
(303) 973-3134

Connecticut

TSA-Connecticut Chapter
(serves entire state)
For current phone number,
contact national TSA.

Association for Children with Learning Disabilities (ACLD)
27 Brainard Rd.
W. Hartford, CT 06117
(203) 233-6191

ACLD State Office
139 N. Main St.
Boatner Bldg.
W. Hartford, CT 06107
(203) 236-3953

Delaware

Tourette Syndrome Association
Delaware Contact
Rt.1, Box 186-1
Hartley, DE 19953
(302) 492-8140

District of Columbia

TSA-Greater Washington Chapter
(serves Maryland, Virginia, and District of Columbia)
For current phone number,
contact national TSA.

District of Columbia Association for Children with Learning Disabilities
1648 Hobart St. N.W.
Washington, DC 20009
(202) 462-0495

Florida

TSA-Florida Chapter
(serves entire state)
For current phone number,
contact national TSA.

Florida ACLD
7016 N. Donald Ave.
Tampa, FL 33614
(813) 637-8957

ACLD
State Office
331 East Henry St.
Punta Gorda, FL 33950
(904) 488-1570

Georgia

TSA of Georgia, Inc.
(serves entire state)
For current phone number, contact national TSA.

Georgia ACLD
3160 Northside Pkwy, NW
Atlanta, GA 30327
(404) 633-5332

ACLD State Office
P.O. Box 29492
Atlanta, GA 30359
(404) 656-2425

Hawaii

Tourette Syndrome Association
Contact: Protection and Advocacy Agency of Hawaii
P.O. Box 15504
Honolulu, HI 96830-5504
(808) 949-2922

Idaho

Idaho ACLD
4610-A Jackson Place
Mountain Home AFB, ID 83648
(208) 832-4218

Illinois

TSA, Inc. of Illinois
(serves entire state)
For current phone number, contact national TSA.

Illinois ACLD
19525 W. Washington
Grayslake, IL 60030
(312) 223-6681, ext. 220

Illinois ACLD
P.O. Box A-3239
Chicago, IL 60690
(312) 663-9535

Indiana

Indianapolis Area TSA
Riley Hospital, Room N-102
702 Barnhill Dr.
Indianapolis, IN 46202-5200
(317) 274-8747

Indianapolis/Central TSA
1017 Oakwood Trail
Indianapolis, IN 46260
(317) 253-8333

Southbend Area TSA
1737 Caroline
Southbend, IN 46618
(219) 234-0671

Iowa

Tourette Syndrome Association
2101 O Avenue, N.W.
Cedar Rapids, IA 52405
(319) 396-0210

Tourette Syndrome Association
112 S.E. Leach
Des Moines, IA 50315
(515) 285-2274

Kansas

TSA-Central Kansas Chapter (serves Colby, Dodge City, Hays, Hutchison, Salina, and Wichita)
For current phone number, contact national TSA.

TSA-Kansas City Chapter
(serves Topeka and Kansas City)
For current phone number, contact national TSA.

Kansas Association for Children with Learning Disabilities
6535 Maple
Mission, KS 66202
(913) 362-9535

Kentucky

TSA-Kentucky Chapter
(serves entire state)
For current phone number, contact national TSA.

Association for Children with Learning Disabilities
Box 13 B
Battletown, KY 40104
(502) 497-4643

ACLD State Office
2232 Alta Ave.
Louisville, KY 40205
(501) 451-8001

Louisiana

Association for Children with Learning Disabilities (ACLD)
8602 Hollow Bluff Dr.
Haughton, LA 71037
(318) 949-2302

Maine

TSA-Maine Chapter
(serves entire state)
For current phone number, contact national TSA.

LDA of Maine
Bessey Ridge Road
Albion, ME 04901
(207) 437-9245

Maryland

TSA-Greater Washington Chapter
(serves Maryland, Virginia, and D.C.)
For current phone number, contact national TSA.

Association for Children with Learning Disabilities
2919 Georgia Ave.
Baltimore, MD 21227
(410) 636-3852

ACLD State Office
320 Maryland National Bank Bldg.
Baltimore, MD 21202
(410) 821-7010
Massachusetts

TSA-Greater Boston Chapter
(serves Boston, Brockton, Buzzards Bay, and Middlesex-Essex)
For current phone number, contact national TSA.

Tourette Syndrome Association
Western MA Chapter
87 Old Farm Rd.
Chicopee, MA 01020
(413) 533-6695

Association for Children with Learning Disabilities
37 Sleigh Rd.
Chelmsford, MA 01824
(508) 256-9598

ACLD State Office
P.O. Box 28
West Newton, MA 02165
(617) 891-5009

Michigan

TSA-Central Michigan Chapter
(serves Flint, Lansing, and Saginaw)
For current phone number, contact national TSA.

TSA-Metropolitan Detroit Chapter
(serves Detroit, Jackson, Kalamazoo, and Royal Oak)
For current phone number, contact national TSA.

TSA-Grand Rapids Chapter
(serves Gaylord, Grand Rapids, Iron Mountain, and Traverse City)
For current phone number, contact national TSA.

Association for Children with Learning Disabilities (ACLD)
8123 E. 9 Mile Road
Big Rapids, MI 49307
(616) 796-8968

Michigan ACLD
P.O. Box 12336
Lansing, MI 48901
(517) 485-8160

Minnesota

TSA-Minnesota Chapter
(serves entire state)
For current phone number, contact national TSA.

Minnesota Association for Children with Learning Disabilities (ACLD)
541 Southwood Dr.
Bloomington, MN 55437
(612) 831-1131

ACLD State Office
1821 University Ave., Room 494-N
St. Paul, MN 55104
(612) 646-6136

Mississippi

Tourette Syndrome Association
181 Rodenberg Ave.
Biloxi, MS 39532
(601) 864-2961

Missouri

TSA-Greater St. Louis Chapter
(serves Cape Girardeau, Flat River, Mid-Missouri Facility Poplar Bluff, Rolla, Sedalia, St. Louis and Springfield)
For current phone number, contact national TSA.

TSA-Kansas City, KS Chapter
(serves Kansas City, St. Joseph, Chillicothe, and Harrisonville)
For current phone number, contact national TSA.

LDA of Missouri
6153 Holmes
Kansas City, MO 64110
(816) 363-5844

LDA State Office
P.O. Box 3302
1918 E. Meadowmere, #10
Springfield, MO 65808
(417) 864-5110

Montana

Tourette Syndrome Association
117 30th Street West
Billings, MT 59102
(406) 652-1883

National TSA

4240 Bell Blvd.
Bayside, NY 11361
(800) 237-0717

Nebraska

TSA-Nebraska Chapter
(serves entire state)
For current phone number, contact national TSA.

Association for Children with Learning Disabilities (ACLD)
5835 Corby
Omaha, NE 68104
(712) 328-8400

Nevada

Tourette Syndrome Association
3201 Pommel Ave.
Las Vegas, NV 89119
(702) 736-8841

New Hampshire

TSA New Hampshire Chapter
(serves entire state)
For current phone number, contact national TSA.

New Hampshire Association for Children with Learning Disabilities
20 Wedgewood Dr.
Concord, NH 03307
(603) 224-5872

New Jersey

TSA of New Jersey, Inc.
(serves entire state)
For current phone number, contact national TSA.

Association for Children with Learning Disabilities (ACLD)
305 North Lancaster Ave.
Margate, NJ 08402
(609) 823-5608

ACLD State Office
640 Ocean Ave.
West End, JN 07740
(201) 229-1919

New Mexico

Tourette Syndrome Association
3301 Montreal, NE
Albuquerque, NM 87111
(505) 291-8591

New York

TSA-Central New York Chapter (serves Elmira, Binghampton, Syracuse, Utica, and Watertown)
For current phone number, contact national TSA.

TSA-Long Island Chapter (serves Nassau and Suffolk Counties, Queens, and the Bronx)
For current phone number, contact national TSA.

TSA-Mid-Western NY Chapter
(serves Rochester)
For current phone number,
contact national TSA.

TSA-New York City West Chapter
(serves Brooklyn, Manhattan,
and Staten Island)
For current phone number,
contact national TSA.

TSA-Westchester/Rockland
County Chapter
(serves Westchester and
Rockland Counties)
For current phone number
contact national TSA.

TSA-Western New York
Chapter
(serves Buffalo and Jamestown)
For current phone number,
contact national TSA.

New York ALD
8 Weiser St.
Glenmont, NY 12077
(518) 783-1644

ALD State Office
90 South Swan St.
Albany, NY 12210
(518) 436-4633

North Carolina

TSA-North Carolina Chapter
(serves entire state)
For current phone number,
contact national TSA.

LDA of North Carolina
510 Colony Woods Dr.
Chapel Hill, NC 27514
(919) 942-1352

LDA State Office
Box 3542
Chapel Hill, NC 27514
(919) 967-9537

North Dakota

North Dakota Tourette Syndrome
Association
3004 Chestnut St.
Grand Forks, ND 53201
(701) 746-7182

Tourette Syndrome Clinic
The Child Evaluation and
Treatment Center
Medical Center Rehabilitation
Hospital and Clinics
Box 8202
Grand Forks, ND 58202
(701) 780-2477

Ohio

TSA of Ohio, Inc.
Park 50 Techne Center
100 Techne Center Dr., Suite 118
Milford, OH 45150

Tourette and Tic Clinic
Ohio State University
Department of Psychiatry
Upham Hall
473 W. 12th Ave.
Columbis, OH 43210
(614) 293-8282

Oklahoma

TSA-Oklahoma Chapter
(serves entire state)
For current phone number,
contact national TSA

Oklahoma Association for
Children and Adults with
Learning Disabilities (ACLD)
1701 Leawood Dr.
Eadmond, OK 73034
(405) 371-2980, ext. 2236

ACLD State Office
3701 N.W. 62nd St.
Oklahoma City, OK 73112
(405) 943-9434

Oregon

TSA-Southern Oregon
Chapter(serves Eugene,
Klamath Falls, and Medford)
For current phone number,
contact national TSA.

Special Education and Student
Services Division
Department of Education
700 Pringle Parkway, S.E.
Salem, OR 97310
(503) 378-3591

Pennsylvania

TSA-South Central Pennsylvania
Chapter (serves Altoona,
Harrisburg, Lancaster,
Lehigh Valley, Philadelphia,
Reading, and Williamsport)
For current phone number,
contact national TSA.

TSA-Northeast Pennsylvania
Chapter (serves Scranton
and Wilks-barre)
For current phone number,
contact national TSA.

TSA-Western Pennsylvania
Chapter (serves Greensburg,
Johnstown, and Pittsburgh)
For current phone number,
contact national TSA.

TSA-Erie Pennsylvania Chapter
(serves Bradford, DuBois,
Erie, New Castle, and Oil City)
For current phone number,
contact national TSA.

Pennsylvania ACLD
2551 W. 8th St.
Erie, PA 16505
(814) 838-1966, ext. 303

ACLD State office
Toomey Building, Suite 23
Eagle, Box 308
Uwichland, PA 19408
(215) 458-8193; (800) 692-6200

Puerto Rico

Puerto Rico ACLD
GPO Box 1905
Sam Juan, PR 00936
(809) 761-0816; (809) 788-6252

Rhode Island

Rhode Island Association for
Children and Adults with
Learning Disabilities (ACLD)
103 Harris Ave.
Johnston, RI 02919
(401) 461-0820, ext. 539

South Carolina

Tourette Syndrome Association
2603 Warren Dr.
Anderson, SC 29621
(803) 224-0683

South Dakota

Tourette Syndrome Association
RR2, Box 93
Parker, SD 57053
(605) 297-4291

Tennessee

TSA-Tennessee State
(serves entire state)
For current phone numbers, contact national TSA.

Tennessee Association for Children and Adults with Learning Disabilities (ACLD)
P.O. Box 114
Pocahontas, TN 38061
(901) 528-6159

Texas

TSA-Dallas/Ft. Worth Chapter (serves Dallas, Ft. Worth, Greenville, Longview, Lufkin, Texarkana, Tyler, and Wichita Falls)
For current phone number, contact national TSA.

TSA-Houston Chapter (serves Beaumont, Bryan, Conroe, Houston, Palestine, Pasadena, and Victoria)
For current phone number, contact national TSA.

TSA-South Central Texas (serves Austin, Corpus Christi, McAllen, San Antonio, Temple and Waco)
For current phone number, contact national TSA.

TSA-South Plains Chapter (serves Abilene, Amarillo, Childress, and Lubbock)
For current phone number, contact national TSA.

Texas Association for Children and Adults with Learning Disabilities (ACLD)
2909 Wildflower
Bryan, TX 77802
(409) 776-2807

ACLD State Office
1011 W. 31st Street
Austin, TX 78705
(512) 458-8234

Utah

TSA-Utah Chapter
(serves entire state)
For current phone number, contact national TSA.

LDA of Utah
2030 E. 9100 St.
Sandy, UT 84093
(801) 943-4425

LDA State Office
P.O. Box 112
Salt Lake City, UT 84110
(801) 364-0126

Vermont

Tourette Syndrome Association
P.O. Box 118
Newfane, VT 05345
(802) 365-4481

TSA Contact
34 Woodlane Apartments
Bristol, VT 05443
(802) 453-3266

TSA Contact
59 Terrill St., Unit #4
Rutland, VT 05701
(802) 747-4436

Virginia

TSA-Greater Washington Chapter
(serves Maryland, Viginia, and District of Columbia)
For current phone number, contact national TSA.

LDA of Virginia
P.O. Box 717
Woodstock, VA 22664
(703) 459-8804

Washington

TSA-Washington State Chapter
(serves entire state)
For current phone number contact national TSA.

LDA of Washington
18921 27th Dr., S.E.
Bothell, WA 98012
(206) 481-8918

LDA State Office
17530 N.W. Union Hill, Suite 100
Redmond, WA 98052
(206) 882-0792

West Virginia

TSA-West Virginia Chapter
(serves entire state)
For current phone number, contact national TSA.

West Virginia Association for Children and Adults with Disabilities (ACLD)
Rt. 3, Box 70
Mineral Wells, WV 26150
(304) 489-9621

Wisconsin

TSA-Wisconsin Chapter
(serves entire state)
For current phone number, contact national TSA.

Wisconsin Association for Children and Adults with Learning Disabilities (ACLD)
2622 Oak Crest Dr.
Neenah, WI 54946
(414) 722-4977

Wyoming

TSA Contact
Box 412
Thermapolis, WY 82443
(307) 864-3603

TSA Contact
P.O. Box 14
Glen Rock, WY 82637
(307) 436-8533

Materials for Parents and Professionals

Hagin, R., Pagano, R., Kreeger, H. (1982). *Effects of Tourette syndrome on learning*. New York: Raven Press.

Haerle, T. (1992). *Children with Tourette syndrome.* Rockville, MD: Woodbine House.

Osman, B. (1982). *No one to play with: The social side of learning disabilities*. New York: Random House.

Rapoport, J. (1989). *The boy who couldn't stop washing: The explanation and treatment of obsessive-compulsive disorder*. New York: Dutton.

Silver, L. (1984). *The misunderstood child.* New York: McGraw-Hill.

Smith, S. (1980). *No easy answers: The learning disabled child at home and at school*. New York: Bantam.

The FCLD Learning Disabilities Resource Guide: *A state by state directory of special programs and services*. New York: The Foundation for Children with Learning Disabilities.

Tourette Syndrome Association. Catalogue of films and brochures. (Available from TSA, 42–40 Bell Blvd., Bayside, NY, 11361.)

APPENDIX D

Resources for Fragile X Syndrome

Organizations

American Association of University Affiliated Programs for Persons with Developmental Disabilities
8605 Cameron Street, Ste. 406
Silver Spring, MD 20910

American Physical Therapy Association
1111 N. Fairfax Street
Alexandria, VA 22314
(703) 684-2782

American Speech-Language-Hearing Association
10801 Rockville Pike
Rockville, MS 20852
(301) 897-5700

The ARC
500 E. Border Street, Ste. 300
Arlington, TX 76010

Autism Society of America
8601 Georgia Avenue, Ste. 503
Silver Spring, MD 20910
(301) 565-0433

Children's Defense Fund
25 E Street N.W.
Washington, DC 20001
(202) 628-8787

Council for Exceptional Children
1920 Association Drive
Reston, VA 22091
(703) 620-3660

Epilepsy Foundation of America
4351 Garden City Drive, Ste. 406
Landover, MD 20785
(800) EFA-1000

Fragile X Southeast Network
Duke University Medical Center
Box 3364
Durham, NC 27710
(800) 654-FRAX

IBM National Support Center for Persons with Disabilities
P.O. Box 2150
Atlanta, GA 30301
(800) IBM-2133
(800) 284-9482 (TDD)

March of Dimes Foundation
1275 Mamaroneck Avenue
White Plains, NY 10605
(914) 428-7100

National Association of Private Schools for Exceptional Children
1522 K Street, N.W., Ste. 1032
Washington, DC 20005
(292) 408-3338

National Association for Visually Handicapped
22 West 21st Street
New York, NY 10010
(212) 889-3141

National Easter Seal Society
70 East Lake Street
Chicago, IL 60601
(312) 726-6200
(312) 726-4258 (TDD)

National Fragile X Foundation
1441 York Street, Ste. 215
Denver, CO 80206
(800) 688-8765
(303) 333-6155

National Information Center for Children and Youth with Disabilities (NICHCY)
P.O. Box 1492
Washington, DC 80206
(703) 893-6061
(800) 695-0285

National Organization on FAS
1815 H. Street, N.W., Ste. 750
Washington, DC 20006

Special Olympics
1350 New York Avenue, N.W., Ste. 500
Washington, DC 20005
(202) 628-3630

Materials

Newsletters and Magazines

The ARC
2501 Avenue J
Arlington, TX 76006

The Exceptional Parent
1170 Commonwealth Ave.
Boston, MA 02134

Pacer Advocate
PACER Center
4826 Chicago Ave S.
Minneapolis, MN 55417

Pacesetter Newsletter
PACER Center
4826 Chicago Ave S.
Minneapolis, MN 55417

Sibling Information Network Newsletter
Connecticut's University Affiliated Program
School of Education
University of Connecticut
Box U-64, Room 227
Storrs, CT 06268

Books

Schopmeyer, B., & Lowe, F. (1992). *The fragile x child*. San Diego, CA: Singular Publishing Group.

APPENDIX E

Resources for Child Neglect/Abuse

Organizations

AMEND
777 Grant Street, Ste. 600
Denver, CO 80203
(303) 832–6363

Association for Children for Enforcement of Support (ACES)
723 Phillips Ave., Ste. 216
Toronto, Ontario
(416) 476–2511

Baltimore Child Abuse Center/Child Advocacy Network
10 South Street, Ste. 502
Baltimore, MD 21202
(410) 396-5165

Child Abuse Institute of Research (CAIR)
P.O. Box 1217
Cincinnati, OH 45201

Child Abuse Listening and Mediation (CALM)
P.O. Box 90754
Santa Barbara, CA 93190–0754
(805) 965–2376

Children's Defense Fund (CDF)
25 E. Street, N.W.
Washington, DC 20001
(202) 628–8787

Clearinghouse on Child Abuse and Neglect Information (CCANI)
P.O. Box 1182
Washington, DC 20013
(703) 385–7565

International Society for Prevention of Child Abuse and Neglect (ISPCAN)
1205 Oneida Street
Denver, CO 80220
(303) 321–3963

National Committee for Prevention of Child Abuse (NCPCA)
332 South Michigan Ave., Ste. 1600
Chicago, IL 60604–4357
(312) 663–3520

National Council on Child Abuse and Family Violence (NCCAFV)
1155 Connecticut Ave., N.W. Ste. 300
Washington, DC 20036
(202) 429–6695

National Institute for Child Support Enforcement (NICSE)
7200 Wisconsin Avenue, Ste 500
Bethesda, MD 20814
(301) 654–8338

National Network of Children's Advocacy Center
(202) 555–1212

People Against Child Abuse
125 Cathedral Street
Annapolis, MD 21401
(410) 296–7816

Voices for Children
10451 Twin Rivers Road
Columbia, MD 21044
(410) 740–0933

APPENDIX F

Resources for Prenatal Drug Exposure

Organizations

Alcohol Helpline
(800) 562-1240

Alcoholism and Substance Abuse Program
Indian Health Service
5600 Fishers Lane
Rockville, MD 20857

Cocaine Baby Help Line
(800) 327-BABE

Fetal Alcohol Education Program
School of Medicine, Boston University
7 Kent Street

Brookline, MA 02146
(617) 739-1424

Healthy Mothers, Healthy Babies Coalition
409 12th Street, S.W. Room 309
Washington, DC 20024
(202) 638-5577
(202) 863-2458

National Association for Perinatal Addiction Research and Education (NAPARE)
11 East Hubbard Street, Ste. 200
Chicago, IL 60611
(312) 329-2512

National Clearinghouse for Alcohol and Drug Information
P.O. Box 2345
Rockville, MD 20852
(301) 468-2600
(800) 729-6686

National Resource Center for Special Needs Adoption
17390 West 8 Mile
Southfield, MI 48075

Materials for Parents and Professionals

Harris, S., & Handelman, S. (Eds.). *Preschool education programs for children with autism*. Austin, TX: Pro-Ed.

Powers, M. *Children with autism: A parent's guide*. Rockville, MD: Woodbine House.

Sacks, O. (1993, December 27). A neurologist's notebook: An anthropologist on Mars. *The New Yorker Magazine*, 106–125.

APPENDIX G

Resources for Autism and Pervasive Developmental Disorder

Organizations

American Speech-Language-Hearing Association
10801 Rockville Pike
Rockville, MD 20852
(800) 638-8255

Autism and Developmental Disabilities Program
UCLA Neuropsychiatric Hospital and Institute
760 Westwood Plaza,

Room C8-720
Los Angeles, CA 90024
(310) 206-7452

Autism Research Institute
4182 Adams Avenue
San Diego, CA 92116
(619) 281-7165

Autism Services Center
605 Ninth Street
Huntington, WV 25710
(304) 206-7452

Autism Society of America
7910 Woodmount Avenue, Ste. 650
Bethesda, MD 20814-3015
(301) 657-0881

Center for the Study of Autism
2207 B Portland Road
Newberg, OR 97132
(503) 538-9045

Eden Institute
One Logan Drive
Princeton, NJ 08540
(609) 987-0099

Exceptional Parent
Psy-Ed Corp.
209 Harvard Street, Ste. 303
Brookline, MA 02146

Indiana Resource Center for Autism
Institute for the Study of Developmental Disabilities
2853 East Tenth Street
Bloomington, IN 47405
(812) 855-6508

International Rett Syndrome Association
8511 Rose Marie Drive
Fort Washington, MD 20744
(301) 248-7031

Sensory Integration International
1402 Cravens Avenue
Torrance, CA 90501-2701
(310) 533-8338

Treatment and Education of Autistic and Related Communication Handicapped Children (TEACCH)
Division of the Department of Psychiatry School of Medicine
CB 7180, 310 Medical School Wing E
The University of North Carolina at Chapel Hill
Chapel Hill, NC 275990-7180
(919) 966-2173

Materials for Parents and Professionals

Dawson, G. (1989). *Autism: Nature, diagnosis, and treatment*. New York: The Guilford Press.

Harris, S. L., & Handleman, J. S. (Eds). (1994). *Preschool education programs for children with autism*. Austin, TX: Pro-Ed.

Powers, M. D. (Ed.). (1989). *Children with autism: A parents' guide*. Rockville, MD: Woodbine House.

APPENDIX H

Assessments for Language Evaluation

Assessment of Children's Language Comprehension (ACLC). Rochana Foster, Jane J. Giddan, & Joel Stark (1983). The Riverside Publishing Company, Chicago, IL.

Bankson-Bernthal Test of Phonology (BBTOP). Nicholas W. Bankson & John E. Bernthal (1990). The Riverside Publishing Company, Chicago, IL.

Bankson Language Test (BLT-2). Nicholas W. Bankson (1990). The Riverside Publishing Company, Chicago, IL.

Carrow Elicited Language Inventory (CELI). Elizabeth Carrow-Woolfolk (1974). The Riverside Publishing Company, Chicago, IL.

Clinical Evaluation of Language, Fundamentals—Revised (CELF-R). Wayne Secord, Eleanor Semel, & Elisabeth H. Wiig (1987). The Psychological Corporation, San Antonio, TX.

Communication Abilities Diagnostic Test (CADeT). Elizabeth B. Johnston & Andrew V. Johnston (1990). The Riverside Publishing Company, Chicago, IL.

Comprehensive Receptive and Expressive Vocabulary Test (CREVT). Gerald Wallace & Donald D. Hammill (1993). The Riverside Publishing Company, Chicago, IL.

Contrast Pairs for Phonological Training. Michael W. Palin (1992). The Riverside Publishing Company, Chicago, IL.

Detroit Test of Learning Aptitude—Primary. Donald D. Hammill & Brian B. Bryant (1986). Pro-Ed, Austin, TX.

Detroit Tests of Learning Aptitude—2 (DTLA-2). Donald D. Hammill (1985). Pro-Ed, Austin, TX.

Expressive One Word Picture Vocabulary Test. Morris F. Gardner (1979). Academic Therapy Publications, Inc., Novato, CA.

Expressive One-Word Picture Vocabulary Test—Revised (EOWPVT-R). Morrison F. Gardner (1990). The Riverside Publishing Company, Chicago, IL.

Expressive One-Word Picture Vocabulary Test—Upper Extension (EOWPVT-UE). Rick Brownell (1983). The Riverside Publishing Company, Chicago, IL.

Fisher-Logemann Test of Articulation Competence. Hilda B. Fisher & Jerilyn A. Logemann (1971). The Riverside Publishing Company, Chicago, IL.

Fluharty Preschool Speech and Language Screening Test. Nancy Buono Fluharty (1968). The Riverside Publishing Company, Chicago, IL.

Fullerton Language Test for Adolescents (FLTA). Arden R. Thorum (1986). The Riverside Publishing Company, Chicago, IL.

Language Sampling, Analysis, and Training (LSAT). Dorothy Tyack & Robert Gottsleben (1974). The Riverside Publishing Company, Chicago, IL.

Of Course I Can. Victoria B. Sperry (1981). The Riverside Publishing Company, Chicago, IL.

Peabody Picture Vocabulary Test—Revised (PPVT-R). Lloyd M. Dunn & Leota M. Dunn (1981). American Guidance Services, Circle Pines, MN.

Porch Index of Communicative Ability in Children (PICAC). Bruce E. Porch (1979). The Riverside Publishing Company, Chicago, IL.

Quick Screen of Phonology (QSP). Nicholas W. Bankson & John E. Bernthal (1990). The Riverside Publishing Company, Chicago, IL.

Receptive One-Word Picture Vocabulary Test (ROWPVT). Morrison F. Gardner (1985). The Riverside Publishing Company, Chicago, IL.

Receptive One-Word Picture Vocabulary Test-Upper Extension (ROWPVT-UE). Morrison F. Gardner (1987). The Riverside Publishing Company, Chicago, IL.

The Receptive-Expressive Emergent Language Scale (REEL)—For the Measurement of Language Skills in Early Infancy. Kenneth R. Bzoch & Richard League (1970). Pro-Ed, Austin, TX.

Revised Token Test. Malcolm M. McNeil & Thomas E. Prescott (1978). Pro-Ed, Austin, TX.

Test for Auditory Comprehension of Language Revised (TACL-R). Elizabeth Carrow-Woolfolk (1985). The Riverside Publishing Company, Chicago, IL.

Test of Adolescent/Adult Word Finding (TAWF). Diane J. German (1990). The Riverside Publishing Company, Chicago, IL.

Test of Adolescent Language (TOAL). Donald D. Hammill, Virginia L. Brown, Stephen C. Larson, & J. Lee Wiederholt (1980). Pro-Ed, Austin, TX.

Test of Adolescent Language (TOAL-3). Donald D. Hammill, Virginia L. Brown, Stephen C. Larsen, & J. Lee Wiederholt (1993). The Riverside Publishing Company, Chicago, IL.

Test of Early Language Development—Revised (TELD-2). Wayne P. Hresko, D. Kim Reid, & Donald D. Hammill (1991). The Riverside Publishing Company, Chicago, IL.

Test of Language Competence-Expanded Edition. Elisabeth H. Wiig & Wayne Secord (1989). The Psychological Corporation, San Antonio, TX.

Test of Language Development (TOLD-2). Phyliss L. Newcomer & Donald D. Hammill (1988). The Riverside Publishing Company, Chicago, IL.

Test of Language Development-Primary; Second Edition (TOLD-P). Phyllis L. Newcomer & Donald D. Hammill (1988). Pro-Ed, Austin, TX.

Test of Nonverbal Intelligence (TONI). Linda Brown, Rita J. Sherbenou, & Susan J. Dollar (1982). Pro-Ed, Austin, TX.

Test of Pragmatic Language (TOPL). Diana Phelps-Terasaki & Trisha Phelps-Gunn (1992). The Riverside Publishing Company, Chicago, IL.

The Test of Pragmatic Skills. Brian B. Shulman (1985). Communication Skill Builders, Tucson, AZ.

Test of Problem Solving. Linda Zachman, Carol Jorgensen, Rosemary Huisingh, & Mark Barrett. LinguiSystems, Inc., Moline, IL.

Test of Word Finding (TWF). Diane J. German (1989). The Riverside Publishing Company, Chicago, IL.

Test of Word Finding in Discourse (TWFD). Diane J. German (1991). The Riverside Publishing Company, Chicago, IL.

Token Test for Children. Frank DiSimoni (1978). The Riverside Publishing Company, Chicago, IL.

Utah Test of Language Development (UTLD-3). Merlin J. Mecham (1989). The Riverside Publishing Company, Chicago, IL.

Weiss Comprehensive Articulation Test (WCAT). Curtis E. Weiss(1980). The Riverside Publishing Company, Chicago, IL.

Woodcock Language Proficiency Battery. Richard W. Woodcock (1980). DLM Teaching Resources, Allen, TX.

Word Finding Referral Checklist (WFRC). Diane J. German (1992). The Riverside Publishing Company, Chicago, IL.

The Word Test, A Test of Expressive Vocabulary and Semantics. Carol Jorgensen, Mark Barrett, Rosemary Huisingh, & Linda Zachman (1981). LinguiSystems, Inc., Moline, IL.

INDEX

A

E

F

O

P

R

S

T

W